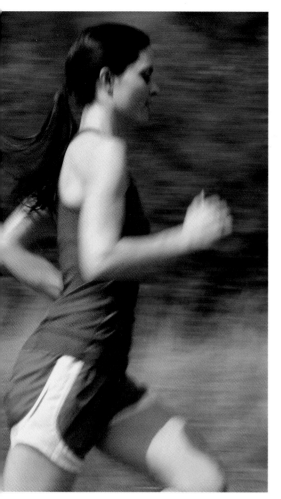

Real Women Run

The complete guide for every female runner

Sam Murphy

Photography by Eddie Jacob

Kyle Books

First published in Great Britain in 2012 by
Kyle Books
an imprint of Kyle Cathie Limited
23, Howland Street
London W1T 4AY
general.enquiries@kylebooks.com
www.kylebooks.com

ISBN: 978 0 85783 009 8

A CIP catalogue record for this title is
available from the British Library

Text © Sam Murphy 2012
Photography © Eddie Jacob 2012, except
p. 79 © John Hicks 2003, p. 137, p. 141,
p. 143, p. 162, p. 169, p. 175, p. 177, p.186,
p. 192, p. 195 © Corbis and p. 196 © Getty
Design © Kyle Books 2012

Editor: Vicky Orchard
Design: Louise Leffler
Photography: Eddie Jacob
Production: Gemma John and Nic Jones
Colour reproduction by Altaimage Ltd
Printed and bound by C & C Offset Printing Co.

Acknowledgements

A big thank you to the many people who helped make this book the
best it could be. I'm so grateful to Jeff Pyrah, Lorraine Western and
Sarah Connors for their invaluable feedback on the text. Thanks also to
Laura Denham-Jones for contributing and starring in the yoga workout,
to Siobhan Burke for additional research and to all the women who
shared their running stories, insights and tips. I'd also like to thank my
lovely group, Rye Runners, for being such obliging models, along with
Holly, Laura, Roberta, Anna and Catherine. Helly Hansen, Nike, Asics
and Vivo Barefoot supplied the fab clothing and footwear. Eddie Jacob
took the pictures.

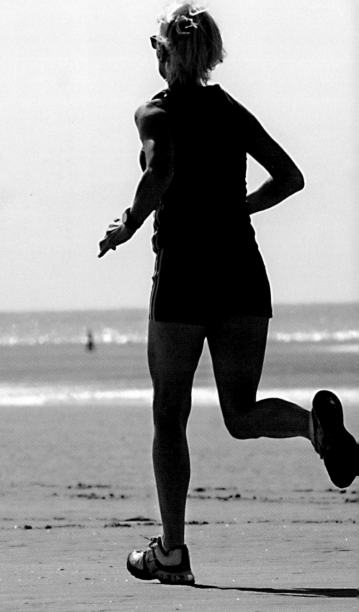

contents

Acknowledgements 2
Introduction 4

Chapter 1: Get inspired 6
Why every woman should run 8
Becoming a runner 16
Claire's story 18

Chapter 2: Starting out 20
Good to go? 22
First steps 25
Getting the habit 33
Annette's story 38

Chapter 3: The essentials 40
Before and after 42
How to run 46

Chapter 4: How to train 56
The rules 58
Your training menu 61
Building a programme 70
On location 74
Helen's story 80

Chapter 5: Balancing act 82
Cross-training 84
Stretch yourself 93
Be strong 98
Staying healthy 110

Chapter 6: The kit list 114
Shoe shop 116
What to wear 122
Training tools 129

Chapter 7: Food and drink 132
Fuel for thought 134
Good hydration 144
Michelle's story 148

Chapter 8: The human race 150
Running together 152
Staying power 157
On your marks 162

Chapter 9: Safe and sound 170
Going solo 172
Damage limitation 174
Running into trouble 178

Chapter 10: Run for life 182
Child's play 184
Teenage kicks 186
Siobhan's story 188
The time of the month 190
Running for two 192
A race against time 198
Sarah's story 202

Resources 204
Index 206

Introduction

Maybe you run purely for the joy of it – you love the breathing space it gives you and couldn't care less about clocking miles or times. Or perhaps it's the challenge of improving your fitness, the sense of accomplishment from achieving new personal bests (PBs). I don't know why you run – or why you are thinking of starting (or restarting), but I do know that you couldn't have picked a better road to health, fitness and happiness. And the aim of this book is to help you on your journey.

Since writing my first women's running book, *Run for Life*, I've accrued nine more years as a runner and coach, qualified as a tutor for UK Athletics, developed my own training workshops, smashed a few PBs and helped dozens of women to achieve their goals (be it a 35-minute 5km or a sub 3 hour 40 minute marathon). As my knowledge and experience have grown, I've found myself marvelling at just how much there is to know about running, and realised there will always be more to learn. That's fine with me – it means there are infinite opportunities to progress.

I can't imagine my life without running. Over the past two decades, it has woven itself seamlessly into my life, having long ago transcended the status of 'workout'. Daily stresses, chores and fears all fade into the background when I set my body in motion. I often find the solutions to problems out on the trail without even searching for them. Running helps me to find focus and clarity or to switch off completely. It can be a tough, challenging pursuit or a gentle, stress-soothing therapy. It can set me up for the day or help me wind down at the end of it. It is my sanctity and my sanity.

But don't get me wrong. I don't train twice a day, wear skimpy shorts, forgo wine and chocolate or run sub-three-hour marathons. My philosophy is for running to enhance my life, not take it over. I want to look good, feel good and protect my health, and running helps me do that. But, like every woman, I have a lot else to fit into

the average day: work, family, social life, household stuff. That's why running is the perfect solution. You can do it any time, with anyone, anywhere. It improves your fitness, health and appearance, and makes you feel better. Come back from a run and you feel alive and ready to take on the world – and win.

You don't need to be athletically gifted to be a runner (and you are still a runner, whether you shuffle round the park twice a week or compete in races worldwide); I never made it into a sports team at school, yet over the past 20 years I have run 15 marathons, innumerable half-marathons, 10km and 5km races, and even dipped my toes into ultra-running (distances greater than the marathon).

While information for female runners isn't the desert it once was (I remember buying one book, written by a man, with a single page on women's running) – many myths and concerns linger. Is it safe to run when you're pregnant? Doesn't running wreck your joints? Is it too late to start running at 50? Do female runners need more iron? Am I fit enough to take part in a race? Is running better than dieting for weight loss? These questions, and many more, are addressed within these pages.

The advice, information and inspiration I offer is gleaned not just from my own years of running and coaching, but from the experiences of other women – from fun runners to elite athletes, newbies to veterans. I've also consulted sport-science experts on everything from footwear to strength training, hydration to motivation, running technique to injury management to ensure that all the information is bang up to the minute. But running is an art as well as a science – and while science provides the map, it's you who creates the path. Whether you want to run 5, 15 or 50km a week, this book will help you to get the most out of every step you take.

Sam Murphy

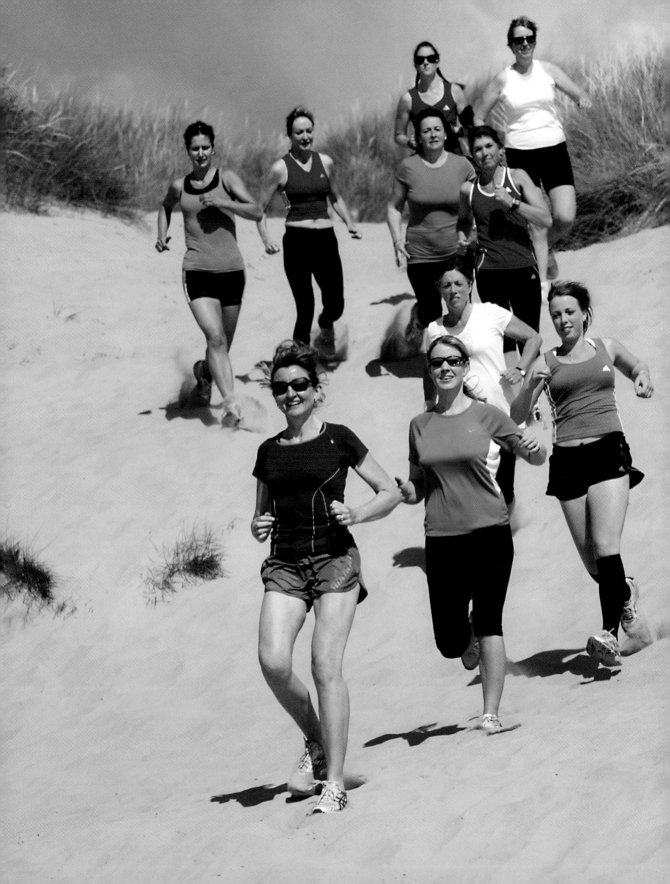

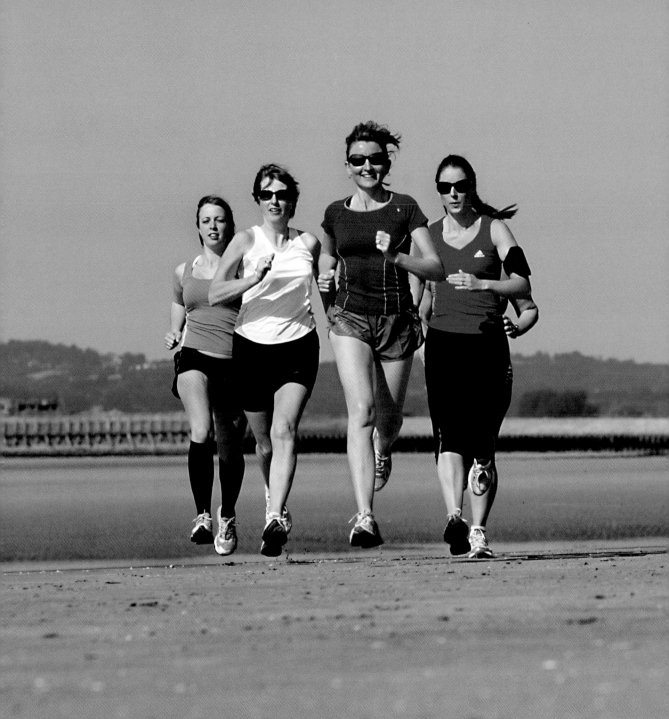

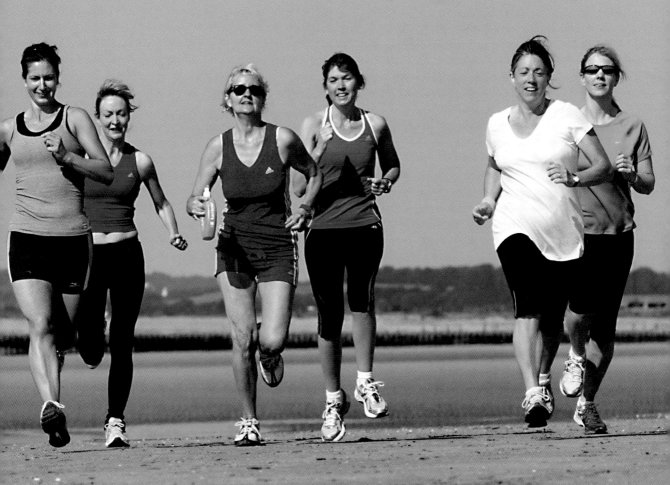

Get inspired

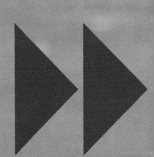

Why every woman should run

Ten reasons to fall in love with running

Why run? Ask a thousand runners that question, and you'll get a thousand different answers. I know women who have run off a broken heart or a stressful week, women who run to escape or to socialise, women who run to lose pounds or to find themselves.

I can never quite remember what made me start running. But whatever it was that got me through those early lung-busting attempts, I'm grateful to it, because my love affair with the sport has become one of my most enduring relationships.

If you are already a runner, you probably have your own answer to 'Why run?' But if you are contemplating starting running, I hope you'll find some convincing reasons to begin over the following pages.

1. It fits your life

Running is convenient, simple and accessible to every woman – even those with lots of juggling to do. Unlike, say, tennis, you don't need to rely on anyone else to play with. Unlike studio classes, you don't need to reserve a place or turn up at a particular time. There's no cumbersome kit or equipment to lug around – and provided you keep a spare pair of trainers in the car, you can go whenever and wherever you like. There's no queue, no fee and the road never closes.

Running is supremely versatile. You can do it alone or with a group, go fast or slow, run for ten minutes or two hours, outdoors or indoors. However you choose to run, you are in control – of the route, the pace, the distance and the amount of effort that you put in. In the time it takes to travel to the gym, work out, get changed and return home you could have completed your run, showered, and launched back into your day with renewed energy.

If you are on a budget, running is one of the cheapest ways of getting and staying fit. It will cost you little more than the price of a decent pair of trainers (see p. 116), unless you kit yourself out with all the latest gear (see p. 122). Heeding the training advice in this book should help you to stay out of the costly sports-injury clinic too.

2. Shed pounds, get toned

As a cardiovascular workout, running outperforms nearly all other exercise. Why? Because you have to carry your own body weight every step. Walking is the same, but one foot is always in contact with the ground, so the workload is easier. In 45 minutes, a 66kg woman burns twice as many calories running at a ten-minute-mile pace compared to walking at a 15-minute-mile tempo. In swimming and cycling, where your weight is supported, energy demand

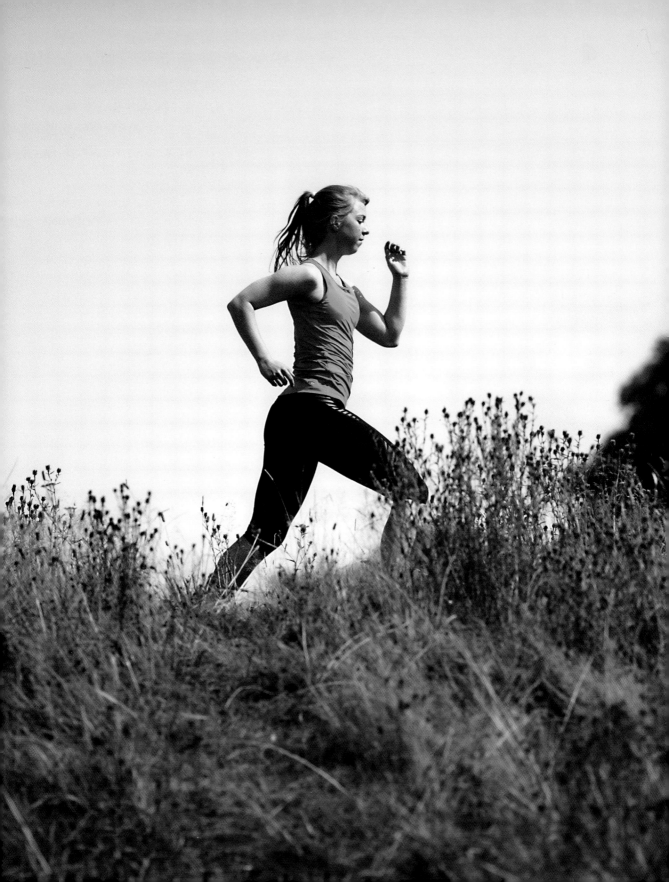

is even lower. Run 10 miles a week and you'll burn approximately 1000 calories – a distance that the *British Medical Journal* reports will reduce your risk of heart disease by a whopping 42 per cent. You'll also firm up every muscle from the waist down and banish the need to watch every calorie you consume. (For more about running and weight loss, see p. 140)

3. A lower risk of breast cancer

Running is fantastic exercise for everyone, but the benefits are particularly compelling when it comes to women's health. Breast cancer is the most common cancer in the UK – affecting 1 in 8 women. While I'd be cautious about stating that running can protect you from breast cancer, there is compelling evidence to suggest that regular physical activity reduces risk. A 2008 study published in the *Journal of the National Cancer Institute* looked at the activity levels of over 60,000 pre-menopausal women: those who did the equivalent of 3.25 hours running per week had a 23 per cent lower risk of breast cancer. Post-menopausal women can also benefit from a more active lifestyle: Polish scientists found women who only took up exercise in their 50s could still slash their breast cancer risk – those in the highest activity category had a 27 per cent risk reduction.

Evidence suggests that regular exercise can protect you from other female cancers too. Research in 2010 found that women who exercise for 150 minutes a week (30 minutes, 5 days a week) have a 34 per cent lower risk of endometrial cancer than inactive women. See Chapter 10 for the impacts on a woman's health throughout her life.

4. Protect your heart

Runners have a lower risk of heart disease. That might sound obvious, but a Harvard Medical School study, spanning two decades, concludes that not only is exercise vital for cardiovascular health, but that more vigorous activities, like running, are more heart-protective than low-to moderate-intensity ones, like walking. A Californian study of 1800 female runners found that their risk of heart

attack was 45 per cent lower than in non-active women. The greater distance the women ran each week the better, but there were benefits even in the lowest mileage group (0–9 miles per week). According to another long-term study, it appears that women experience greater heart health-boosting benefits from exercise than men. While running has a positive effect on resting heart rate, blood pressure, body-fat levels and HDL ('good' cholesterol) in both sexes, only in women do 'bad' LDL cholesterol levels significantly decrease – especially post-menopause. Such a boost is valuable at any age, but post-menopause it is imperative. This is when the heart-protective effects of oestrogen disappear, increasing a woman's risk of heart disease. Chapter 10 has more information on how running can help you grow old gracefully.

5. Get smarter

Your brain also benefits from regular workouts. A 2009 University of Gothenburg study of more then 1 million people, found a clear link between high levels of physical fitness and better results in an IQ test. Aerobic fitness was connected to improvements in logical thinking and verbal comprehension, making running the ideal workout for a brain boost. It's thought that enhanced oxygen flow to the brain stimulates mental function.

It's never too late to benefit – a 2010 University of Washington School of Medicine study showed women aged 55–85 with mild cognitive impairment who exercised vigorously, four days a week, improved on measures of mental function (like recalling a story or learning a list) more than women who undertook low-intensity exercise over a six-month period.

6. Boost body confidence

Negative body image affects us all – 60 per cent of people claim to be dissatisfied with their appearance – but the problem has been described as epidemic among women. We're surrounded by images of stick-thin women in magazines or on TV as if they are the norm, and women can feel like failures for not being a size 10 (let alone a size zero!). But active women don't seem to suffer such a high degree of body dissatisfaction. And it's not just because they have better bodies. Research from the University of Florida in 2009, which reviewed over 50 studies on body image and exercise, found that exercise is enough to make people feel more confident about their appearance, whether they become fitter or not. Running is one of the best ways of tuning into the physical side of your body, as it is so simple and focused. Progress is easily measured, allowing you to experience success through using your body – a boon to self-esteem, body image and confidence. Run outside and you'll avoid any self-criticism in the mirror too.

Feeling better about your body can have some unexpected pay-offs: a 2004 University of Arkansas study found that people who exercise perceive themselves as more sexually desirable and experience greater levels of sexual satisfaction.

7. Bone up

Contrary to popular belief, running does not 'wreck your knees' or wear out your joints. Stanford University monitored 500 runners and 500 non-runners over a 20-year period and found that the non-runners had suffered more, not less, wear and tear on their joints. While bone density begins to decrease from around the age of 35 (with depletion speeding up post-menopause) high-impact activities, such as running, increase bone density more effectively than low-impact ones like swimming, because putting bone under stress is what makes it adapt and grow stronger. A study in *Osteoporosis International* found that masters runners (over 65 years old) had significantly greater bone mineral density than masters swimmers and non-athletes. Around 3 million people in the UK suffer from osteoporosis, with 1 in 3 women over the age of 50 suffering an osteoporotic fracture – usually at the hip, wrist or spine. It's well worth fortifying your bones; read more about how to protect yourself in Chapter 10.

8. Don't worry, be happy

Running is a great stress release – you nearly always return from a run feeling calmer and more focused. According to research from Boston University, people who exercise report fewer symptoms of anxiety and depression, and lower levels of stress and anger. The positive effect of exercise on stress is usually attributed to endorphins – neurotransmitters that give us a 'euphoric' feeling. But the

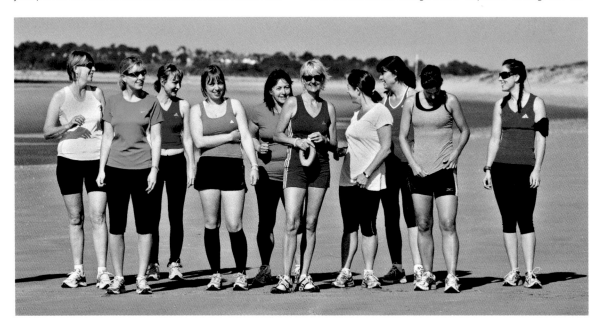

> "The greatest benefit of running is realising that I have the power and ability to make visible, tangible changes to my body and fitness. At school I used to skive off PE when we had the 1500m as I 'knew' I wouldn't be able to run that far. I'm not a natural long-distance runner, so it has been really gratifying to see what can be achieved with persistence and sheer bloody-mindedness – for me, a sub-two-hour half marathon."
>
> Clare

1–2kg over subsequent decades. This is partly down to changes in metabolism as we age, but, increasingly, scientists believe it is because we become less active as we get older, lowering our energy expenditure and causing calorie-hungry muscle mass to decline. A less active lifestyle also leads to reduced joint mobility and stiffer muscles. But research from Tel Aviv University shows that regular exercise increases what's known as 'spontaneous locomotion' – the instinct that makes us want to 'get up and dance', which typically declines with ageing. In other words, the more you move, the more you'll want to move! Find out why running is the perfect anti-ageing sport in Chapter 10.

10. Live longer

Running doesn't just add life to your years – it can also add years to your life. According to the American College of Sports Medicine's 2009 study, regular exercise can increase life expectancy and delay the onset of chronic disease and disabling conditions, such as heart disease, diabetes, obesity, arthritis and osteoporosis. Any form of physical activity is good, but research in the *Journal of Science and Medicine in Sport* found that runners live between 2.8 and 5.7 years longer than the general population.

So what's stopping you?

Healthier, slimmer, fitter, smarter, happier ... What are you waiting for? If this is the point at which you would normally reel off your long list of excuses as to why running isn't your thing, read on.

'I'm too unfit to start'

Every journey begins with a single step. It's an old cliché, but it's true. I know women who could barely run for a couple of minutes who have now completed half marathons. But you have to be patient and start slowly. Doing too much, too soon is the most common beginner's mistake and a sure way to put yourself off before you've got started. The best advice is to run as much as you can

act of distraction from worries is undoubtedly a factor too.

The Boston researchers are so convinced by the benefits of exercise that they recommend it be prescribed as an alternative to prescription drugs for anxiety and depression. Just 25 minutes of aerobic exercise is enough to improve your mood and boost energy. The social aspect of exercise can also play a role in combating depression, so if you're feeling blue, consider running in a group or with a friend. See chapter 8 to find out more.

9. Look and feel younger

Getting fit can help combat many of the effects of ageing. Increased oxygen and blood flow to the skin improves its appearance and tone, while perspiration allows toxins to be released, giving a youthful glow. The average person typically gains 8–9kg of body weight (mostly fat) between the ages of 18 and 55, followed by additional gains of and walk as much as you need. You'll be amazed how quickly you are able to build up your running. And don't give that whippet-thin bloke overtaking you in the park a second thought – he's probably been at it for years – and anyway, he's just trying to impress you! There's loads more information for newbie runners in Chapter 2.

'It's boring'

Anyone who believes that running is boring has missed the point. Running the same route, at the same pace, day after day, might be boring, but that's no more necessary than eating the same meal every evening. Running can be anything to anyone. The secret to making a lifelong commitment to running is to keep it varied, fun and challenging so you'll continue to reap results without succumbing to boredom or burnout. You can learn more about setting goals and creating a balanced training programme later in the book.

'I'm not competitive'

Many women shy away from the idea of racing, shuddering at unpleasant memories of competitive sports at school. But there's no need to get involved in competitive running unless you want to – improving on your own efforts is challenging enough. Running can be competitive but, rest assured, many people enjoy running without ever completing a race. That said, in my experience, many women who say they aren't competitive are fiercely so. They just haven't yet unleashed it! Read more about choosing the right race for you in Chapter 8.

'It's too embarrassing'

If you think everyone will look at you when you run, think again. People are too wrapped up in their own lives to give you more than a passing glance. If you are really concerned about being heckled or laughed at, get some moral support by running with a friend or running group. If you prefer – or need – to run alone, then go out early, before anyone else is up, avoid busy areas and head off the beaten track (although check out my safety tips on p. 172).

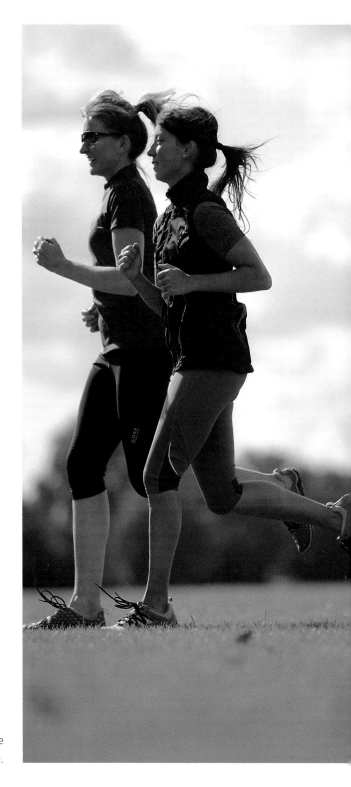

As a last resort, there's always the treadmill, if you feel too embarrassed to run in the great outdoors – although I recommend viewing this as temporary, until you build confidence, rather than as a long-term solution.

'I'm too old'

I don't know how old you are, so I can't state that you are, or are not, too old to start running. But unless you have a degenerative joint or bone condition (such as osteoarthritis or osteoporosis), a heart, lung or other serious health problem, there is no reason to rule out running. Even in some of the above circumstances, running can be a safe and enjoyable exercise, provided you have medical clearance. Older runners do need to be wiser runners – taking more recovery between sessions and being more vigilant about warming up – but you can reap health gains from running at any age.

'I'm overweight'

Runners come in all shapes and sizes. A few extra kilograms should not stand between you and running. Rather than taking the 'I better lose some weight first' approach, why not give running a try? This is a proactive strategy that helps you lose weight from day one, rather than waiting until the latest 'miracle' diet works. In a 2009 Cuban study, overweight and obese women assigned to thrice-weekly jogging sessions for eight weeks achieved weight loss, improved cholesterol profile, lowered blood pressure and reduced waist–hip ratio. If you are significantly overweight (see p. 23), you need to take extra care that you aren't putting too much stress on your body – which means it may be preferable to start with walking, gradually introducing small amounts of running, which you can increase as you feel able. I know many women who have begun this way and lost substantial amounts of weight at the same time as falling in love with running.

'I haven't got time'

This excuse tops them all. Running is one of the fastest

I took up running after having children; it helped me regain my fitness fast. It's easy to fit in, it doesn't take long and it's on your doorstep, unlike many gyms. As a mother of three, running gives me my own space, away from everything else and leaves me feeling full of energy.

Minna

ways to exercise – and with minimal preparation. Even 15 minutes will energise, tone and strengthen and burn calories. If you think you don't have time to run, there is little hope that you will manage any other exercise.

The funny thing about time is that we all have the same amount. It's how we use it that differs and when it comes to something as important as your health (not to mention your waistline and mood), it's about *taking* time, not making time, for running. In one 2009 study, 85 per cent of women who claimed they didn't have time to exercise spent more than an hour a day of their free time in front of the TV or computer. For advice on how to fit running into your lifestyle see page 33.

Raring to go? Whether you've never run a step, are itching to make the transition from treadmill to trail or simply lost your running mojo and want to try again, read on to find out how to become the runner you want to be.

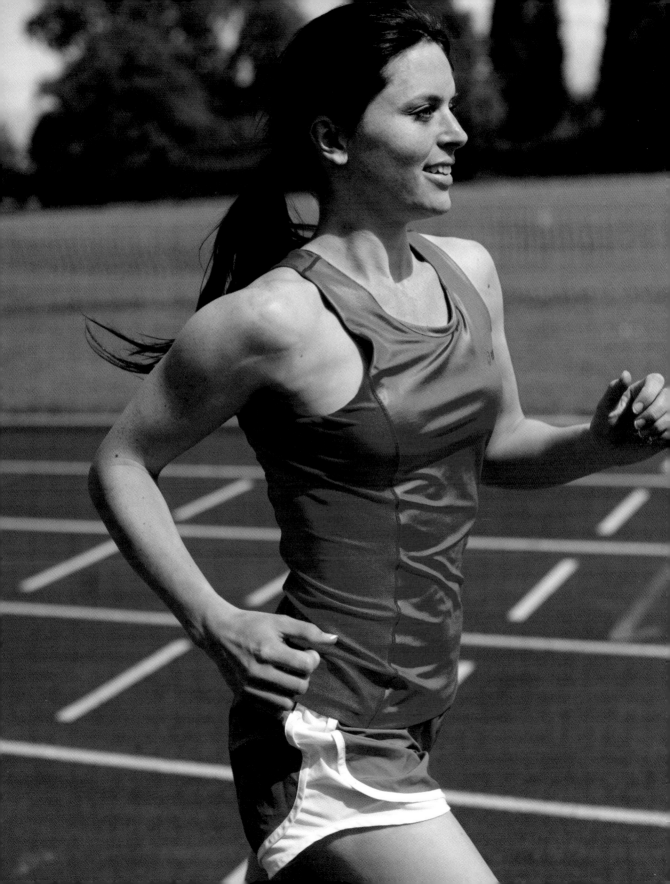

Becoming a runner
How your body gets fitter

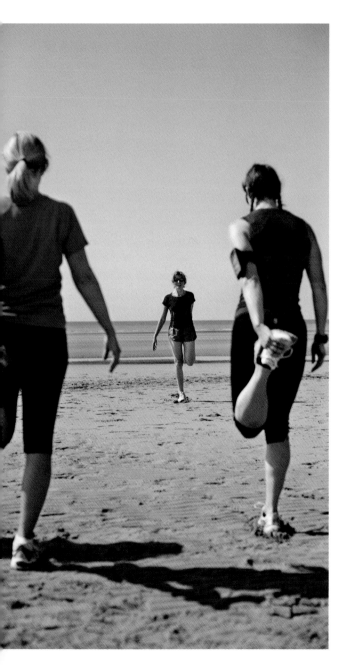

The body is an amazing machine. Its capacity for improvement and adaptation means that something that might seem inconceivable – such as running a marathon, 5km or to the end of the road – is within your grasp, if you build up slowly, but surely. While you might think it likes sitting on the sofa, your body actually likes being challenged; the challenge triggers the changes that make you fitter, slimmer and healthier. Here's how it works.

When you start running, your heart rate (the number of times it beats per minute – bpm) and stroke volume (the amount of blood pumped out by your heart with each beat) go up. Why? Because your previously resting muscles now have to do some work, for which they need lots of oxygen. Blood (red blood cells, in particular) acts as the courier for oxygen (as well as other nutrients) around the body, so the heart has to pump harder and faster to supply the muscles' needs and to meet the new energy demand. The amount of oxygenated blood that flows from the heart every minute is called your cardiac output.

Increased cardiac output is one of the most important adaptations that result from training. As your heart gets stronger, it can pump out more blood per minute, reducing the beats needed to deliver the same amount of oxygen. So resting heart rate drops as you get fitter, while stroke volume increases. If running a ten-minute mile took your heart rate up to 160bpm before, the same pace might elevate it to 150bpm after a few weeks of regular training. To get your heart rate back up to 160bpm you would need to run faster. The great thing is, it won't feel any harder, as your fitness will have increased. This is called 'running economy' – I like to think of it as your 'miles per gallon' rate. The more economical you are, the less effort it will take to sustain any pace.

The blood arrives at the muscles through a network of tiny capillaries, which are flimsy enough to allow oxygen and nutrients to pass through (and carbon dioxide and waste products to exit). The muscle picks up oxygen from the blood, dumps some carbon dioxide, and the blood returns to the heart. But – and it's a big but – the muscle cell isn't able to take all the oxygen that the blood is carrying; it can only take some of it. Your muscle cells' capacity to extract oxygen from blood is a crucial factor in running. It's no good having oxygen-rich blood flowing to the muscles if they can collect only a tiny proportion of it. The good news is that regular running increases the number of capillaries in the muscle, creating a larger surface area for oxygen to be absorbed. The average person has three to four capillaries per muscle fibre, whereas a well-trained runner might have five to seven. The runner's oxygen extraction is far superior because the oxygen-rich blood 'hangs around' the muscle cell longer while travelling through the capillaries, giving more time to pick up the oxygen.

The maximum rate at which oxygen can be extracted from the air, transported by the blood and used by the muscles is called your maximal oxygen uptake, or VO_2 max. It has long been considered the 'gold standard' of aerobic fitness. Your VO_2 max is partly determined by gender (women have a lower VO_2 max than men), genetics and age, but it will almost certainly increase as you run regularly. Training can result in improvements from 5 to 25 per cent. A sedentary woman might have a VO_2 max of 30ml/kg/min (kg referring to her body weight), while a well-trained woman might be closer to 60ml/kg/min.

But what's the big deal about all this oxygen? It's all to do with energy production. When enough oxygen flows through the blood to meet energy needs, the 'powerhouses' of the muscle cells (the mitochondria) can use that oxygen to produce energy from the breakdown of a substance called adenosine triphosphate (ATP). Since the body can only store enough ATP to last for a couple of seconds, it needs to be broken down continuously to sustain any activity. When there isn't enough oxygen to meet demand, the muscle cells have to make ATP without oxygen or 'anaerobically'. This is far less efficient for an endurance activity like running because it results in the accumulation of lactic acid and a build-up of hydrogen ions, which makes the muscle very acidic and hampers muscular contraction. The lactic acid is removed, but if it is produced at a faster rate than it can be eliminated, it builds up in the muscle and, before you know it, you've crossed the 'lactate threshold' (sometimes called the anaerobic threshold). The lactate threshold is the point at which lactate clearance cannot keep up with lactate production, causing a sharp rise in the level in the blood. Beyond it, you feel your lungs are fit to burst, your legs are like concrete and your brain's screaming 'Stop!'

When you are new to running, you can reach this point pretty soon. But as you get fitter, your aerobic capacity will improve, pushing the threshold point closer to your VO_2 max and allowing you to work at higher intensities without it feeling so tough. There is no genetic component to lactate threshold – so you can keep on raising it and reaping the benefits of working harder and longer. Find out more in chapter 4.

Several factors play a part in this change, including an increase in the number and size of mitochondria. You'll even increase the amount of blood in your body.

Another bonus of regular aerobic training is that it teaches the body to use fat as its energy source, instead of carbohydrate. This is good news not just because utilising fat means you'll have less of it clinging to your thighs (not to mention your heart), but also because it allows glycogen, the body's carbohydrate stores, to be 'spared'. Glycogen is the body's preferred fuel source, and since we only have limited storage capacity, it's good to preserve it where possible, and use fat, which is usually available in unlimited supply! To make things even more efficient, your glycogen stores will expand through training – studies show increases of up to 40 per cent.

These changes take place from your first steps as a runner and, as long as your training is smart and consistent, they keep on coming.

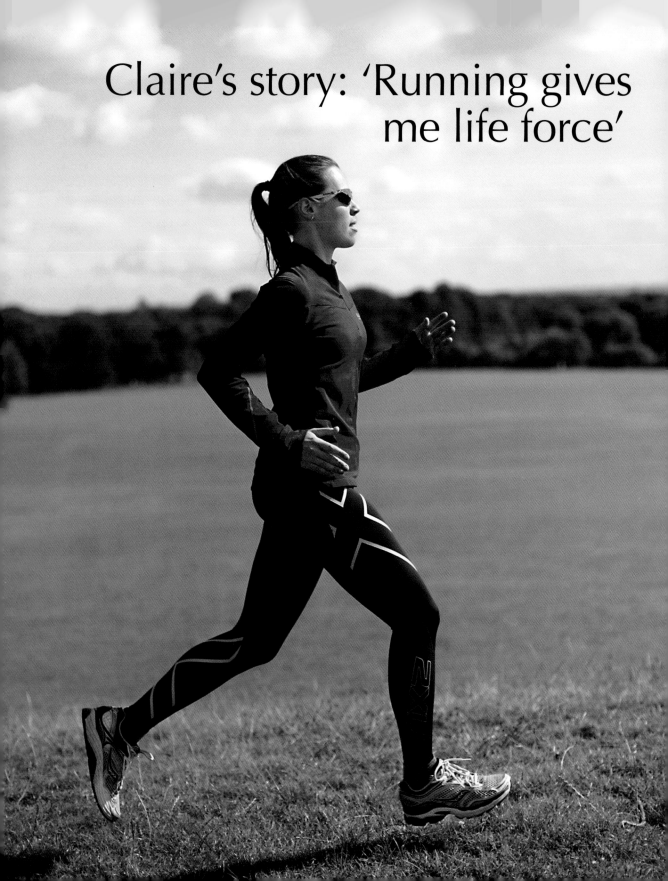

Claire's story: 'Running gives me life force'

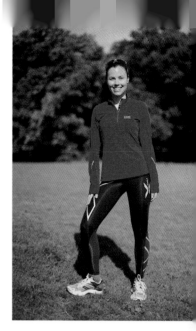

"

It was a broken heart that motivated me to start running. I had moved to London to be with the man I'd fallen in love with whilst travelling through South America – but a year later, our relationship came to an end. Although the break-up was amicable, I was nonetheless devastated and needed a healthy challenge to drive me out of my hole and rediscover parts of myself that I had long neglected.

One morning, an ad for the Royal Parks Half Marathon caught my eye. Although I hadn't run regularly for years and had never run more than six miles, I signed up. I felt a rush of excitement, and then one of fear. How could I successfully juggle an intensive running plan with myriad other things vying for my time?! Initially, I struggled to find the right balance between prioritising my training and, for example, staying late at work to finish an urgent project, going on a date, helping my sister plan her wedding, spending a weekend in Istanbul…However, I quickly discovered that running doesn't take time – it gives life force. With each step, I was both clawing back my old self and building the foundation for a new, improved version.

Fittingly, as I had taken up running to leave my previous relationship behind, I did just that on race day – both literally and figuratively. I not only recovered from my emotional slump but also smashed my first half marathon to pieces, beating my ex (who also happened to be competing) by four minutes! He was proud of me, but visibly annoyed, which made victory that much sweeter.

Perhaps it isn't a surprise that my passion for running ultimately sparked my current romance. I was at a party, chatting about training for my first marathon, when another runner joined the conversation. It was refreshing to finally connect with someone who shared my love of running! We dated for several months, and after I had completed the Paris marathon – aided by his support and encouragement – my gut confirmed that he was the right guy. Seven months later, we both finished the NYC marathon – his first, and my first sub-3:40. I was incredibly grateful not only to have achieved my goal, but also to celebrate with someone I love who understood exactly how I felt, down to waking up the next morning and hardly being able to hobble to the bathroom!

As time goes on, running continues to inspire me – as I coast along the river before the Monday morning rush; as I furiously attack an interval session prior to an important meeting; as I chat breathlessly with a running buddy in between hill repeats; as I shift gears in mile 16 towards a well-earned Sunday pancake breakfast; as I savour a refreshing breeze along a stretch of beach in Zanzibar; or as I sprint across a finish line and realise – I did it.

What is consistent across all of these runs is that powerful, uplifting feeling of endorphins coursing through my body, translating into the confidence, courage and positive energy that fuel the rest of my day – or dare I say, life.

"

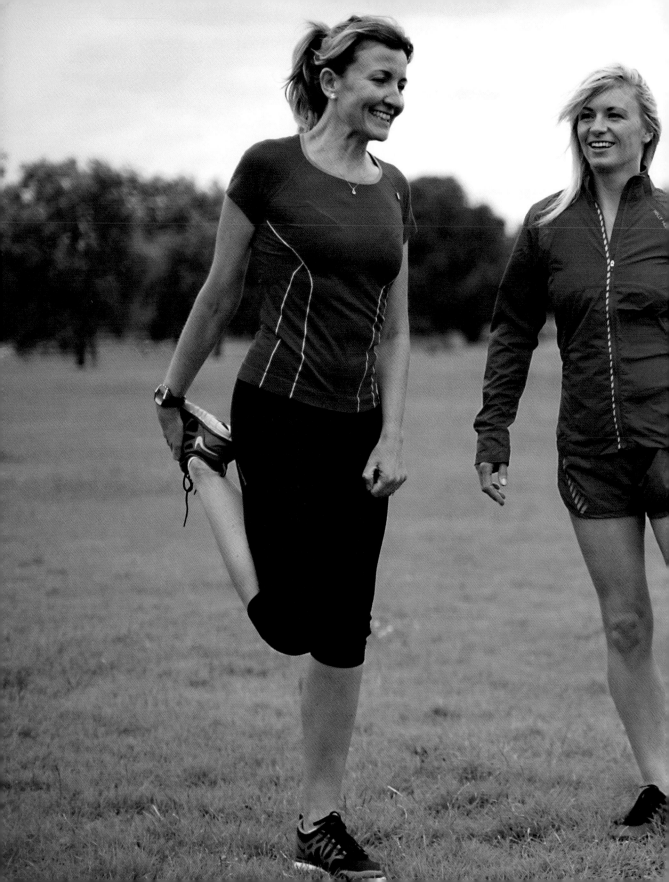

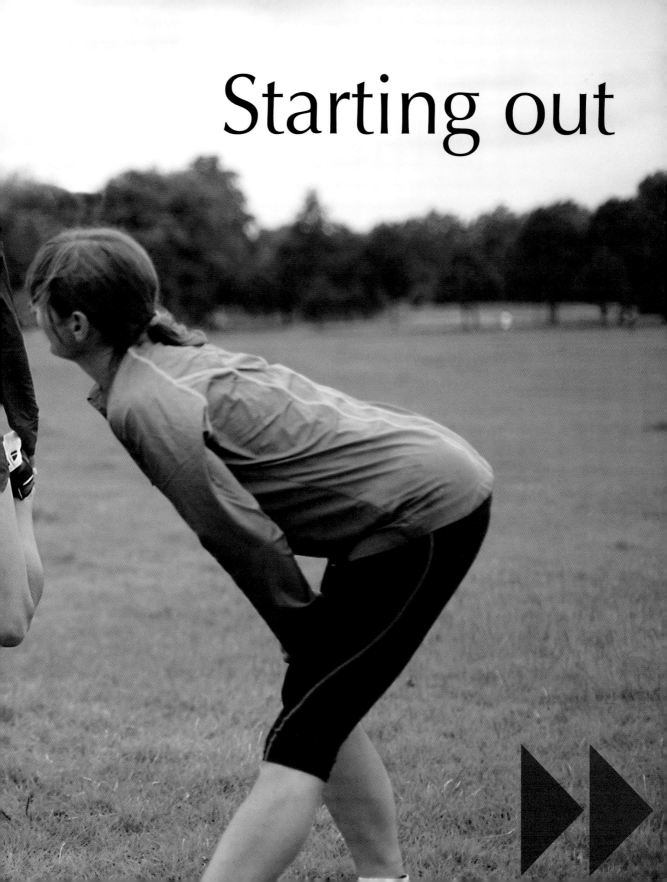

Starting out

Good to go?
Getting off on the right foot

You don't need to be super-fit to start running but following the training advice in this book will allow your body to adapt without undue stress, pain or risk. There are, however, a few factors that may affect your suitability for running. Consider these questions carefully to see if you should seek medical advice before beginning.

- Have you ever been diagnosed with a heart condition by your doctor?
- Do you experience chest pain during physical activity?
- In the past month, have you had chest pain when you were not doing physical activity?
- Do you lose your balance because of dizziness, or do you ever lose consciousness?
- Is your BMI higher than 30 (see opposite page)?

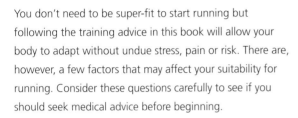

- Do you have a bone or joint problem (such as osteoarthritis or osteoporosis) or an injury that could be made worse by a change in your physical activity?
- Are you currently taking medication for high blood pressure or a heart condition, or is your blood pressure higher than 140/90?
- Are you pregnant or have you recently had a baby? (See p. 192 for more information.)
- Do you have a parent or sibling who has or had premature heart disease (in men under 55 or women under 65)?
- Do you believe there are any other reasons why running may negatively affect your health?

If you answered 'Yes' to any of these questions, you should consult your doctor before running or continuing with your existing exercise programme. If you are a woman over 55, or have done no exercise for more than a year, you may want to get the all-clear from your doctor before starting to run, even if your answers are all 'No'.

If you answered 'No' to all the questions, you are ready to start running. First things first:

- If you are suffering from an injury, pain, or illness of any kind, delay starting until it has been addressed.
- If you have suffered musculoskeletal injuries in your back or legs or have any kind of postural or biomechanical abnormalities (such as a scoliosis or a leg length discrepancy), it's worth being assessed by a physiotherapist or podiatrist before you begin running.
- If you cannot walk briskly for 30 minutes comfortably, spend the next three to four weeks working up to this goal before starting the beginner's programme on p. 28.

Running and body mass index (BMI)

If you are overweight and unsure whether running will be healthy for you, calculate your BMI. If it is over 30, you should consider starting with something less impactful than running to avoid putting your body under undue stress, or aim to lose some weight before starting. BMI is a way of assessing healthy body weight – taking into account weight and height. It's not an exact science though – if you are muscular, you may have a higher BMI, because muscle weighs more than fat. For the same reason, it's not a good measure of progress because as you get fitter, your body replaces fat with muscle, so you may look trimmer, but be heavier. Do the calculation, but remember it's just a guideline.

Calculating your BMI

Measure your height in metres and your weight in kilograms, then divide your weight by your height squared. The ideal range is 18.5–24.9. Don't worry too much if your BMI is below 18.5, as long as you are in good health (and, if pre-menopausal, are having regular periods).

Below 18.5	underweight
18.5–24.9	optimal range
25–29.9	overweight
30+	very overweight

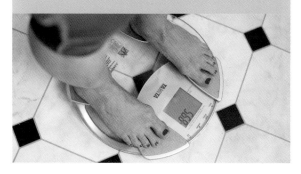

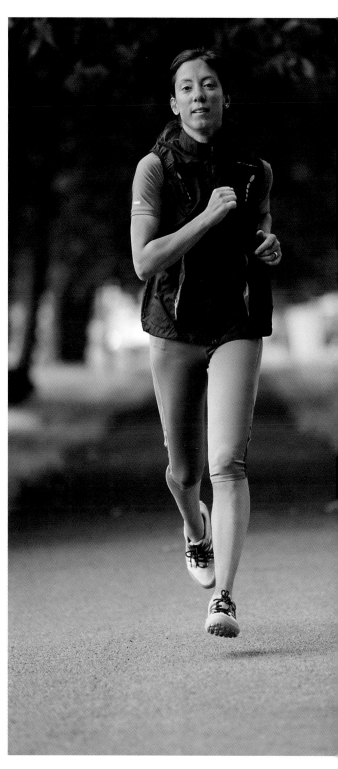

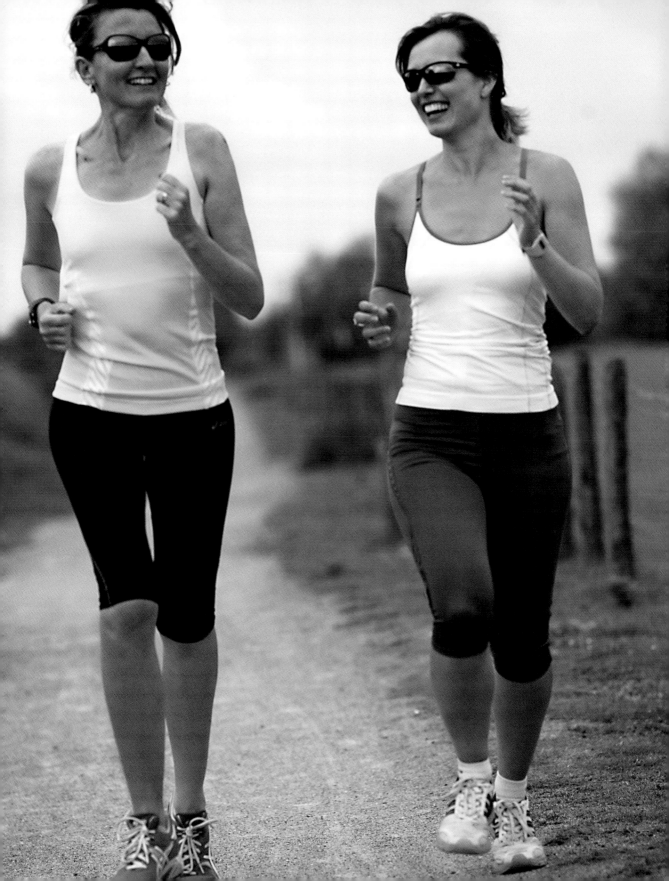

First steps
Advice for new runners

Aside from decent trainers and a sports bra, the most important attribute for a new runner is the right attitude. Rather than something to be mastered or conquered, I see running as a voyage of discovery – where the journey is just as important as the destination. Whatever your reason for taking up running – to lose weight, de-stress or run a certain distance – you'll find many more reasons to keep it up. I've been running for over two decades and I'm still finding new things to learn and enjoy. Like any good investment, it just keeps on giving!

In my experience, many new runners expect too much, too soon and give up or get injured before they've enjoyed the benefits. If you're taking up running after a long period of inactivity, remember how long it took to get out of shape – you're not going reverse things overnight. And nor should you want to.

Seeing running as a lifelong habit, rather than as a quick fix, helps you to reap far more benefits from it – new friendships, personal goals, confidence, fun – as well as fewer negatives, such as injury, frustration, fatigue.

And if you stick with running, you can expect to improve more than an Olympic athlete. You might not match their achievements as far as speed goes, but because elite athletes operate so near their genetic potential, they have to work really hard to gain tiny improvements. The rest of us, somewhat further away from our genetic ceilings, can expect to progress exponentially – and no more so than during the first few months.

Slowly but surely

My favourite phrase for new runners is 'make haste slowly'. That means not trying to progress too fast, in terms of your running pace and how quickly you increase the length of your runs. These are the most common beginner mistakes, and the ones most liable to result in you giving up because it's too hard, feeling disillusioned because you haven't advanced as much as you thought you would or, worst of all, getting injured. Here are my four golden rules for making haste slowly:

1. Run slower than you think you can

The way to become a runner isn't to go as fast as you can for as long as you can before collapsing. The key is finding a pace that, for you, feels comfortable and achievable and, most importantly, sustainable for a meaningful period of time. We call this 'conversation' pace – the pace at which you could chat to a friend: if you can barely utter two words to your jogging buddy, you're working too hard; if you can yak non-stop, you are taking it a bit too easy. A good guideline is that you should be getting warm and slightly breathless. You'll find that you will be able to increase your pace without increasing your effort level as your body adapts to the challenge of running.

To begin with, focus on how long you can run for, not how fast. The target is to get to the point where you can run continuously, however slowly, for 30 minutes or so without needing to stop or walk. It's only once you are comfortable with this that you should start experimenting with pace.

2. Walk as much as you need to

Run as much as you can, then walk as much as you need to while you recover and get your breath back. Then repeat, repeat, repeat. As the weeks progress, you'll be able to run for a little longer each time.

The beginners' programme on p. 28 is based on a 'walk–run' strategy. I've found that this is the best way for beginners to ease themselves into running – many have progressed within weeks to completing a 5km race.

Please do not see walking as a failure, or as a poor substitute for running. It's far smarter to intersperse walking and running bouts from the outset of a session than to stick to running but have to cut your workout short. If you don't believe me, consider the following example:

Anna (who weighs 10 stone 7lb) can run continuously for seven minutes (at a 10-minute-mile pace). In those seven minutes, she'll burn 78 calories. But if she were to intersperse each minute of running with two minutes of brisk walking, she'd extend her workout to a much more meaningful total of 23 minutes and burn 167 calories. And once she can up the running to two minutes per bout, her energy expenditure goes up to 245 calories.

3. Do not run every day

Running every day is not necessary – indeed, when you're starting out, it's better not to. Take a day off between each running session – maintaining consistency without overdoing things. You don't have to do nothing on 'off' days; but stick to low-impact exercise, like strength training, or non-impact, like swimming, to give your joints a break and allow them to adjust to the forces of running. This obeys the 'hard–easy' rule (which you'll read more about in Chapter 4) – following your toughest training days with easier runs or rest days. Coaches use this to ensure runners get a balance of hard work and recovery.

4. Take baby steps

Don't try to progress too quickly – a sharp increase in mileage is a prime cause of injuries. You may have a good level of fitness from a different aerobic activity, like cycling or swimming, but you need to allow your body time to adapt to running's unique demands – in particular, the impact on your muscles, joints and bones (the musculoskeletal system). Even if you feel like you could advance your training quite substantially, do not increase by more than around 10 per cent per week. For example, if you did three miles, four times a week (a total of 12

miles), you could up it to 13.2–13.5 miles the following week. If measuring your runs by time, the same rule applies; if you ran for 30 minutes, four times a week (120 minutes), you could increase your total by 12 minutes the following week. It's also important to have the odd easier week where you don't up your training at all. For more on constructing a balanced training programme see Chapter 4.

0–20 in eight weeks

The eight-week beginners' programme on pages 28–29 is designed to get you to the point at which you can run continuously for 20 minutes. It is based on training four days per week, mixing bouts of running with walking to reduce the amount of stress you are placing on your musculoskeletal system (which won't yet be accustomed to the impact of running).

Start each run with a warm-up to prepare your body and leave time for a cooldown, which allows your heart rate and breathing rate to return to normal (read how to warm up and cool down in Chapter 3). Then stretch the muscles that you have worked (see the runner's stretch in Chapter 5).

The ideal surface for running is level trail or grass – it's more forgiving than concrete, but not so unstable that it will compromise your technique. An athletics track is another option. It isn't always possible to avoid running on pavements or roads – so don't worry if that's all that is available. Once your runs take you further, you will find a greater variety of surfaces. You could do some of your running on a treadmill, but try not to become too reliant on it – it's not quite the same as running in the 'real world'.

Try to run on a fairly flat surface. Hills have their place, but for now, the aim is to make everything as easy as possible. If you do encounter a hill, think about maintaining the same effort level as on the flat (let your pace slow down, so you don't end up fighting for breath).

I know it's a big commitment to run four days a week, but I highly recommend you incorporate some strength and stability exercises to work on your core muscles.

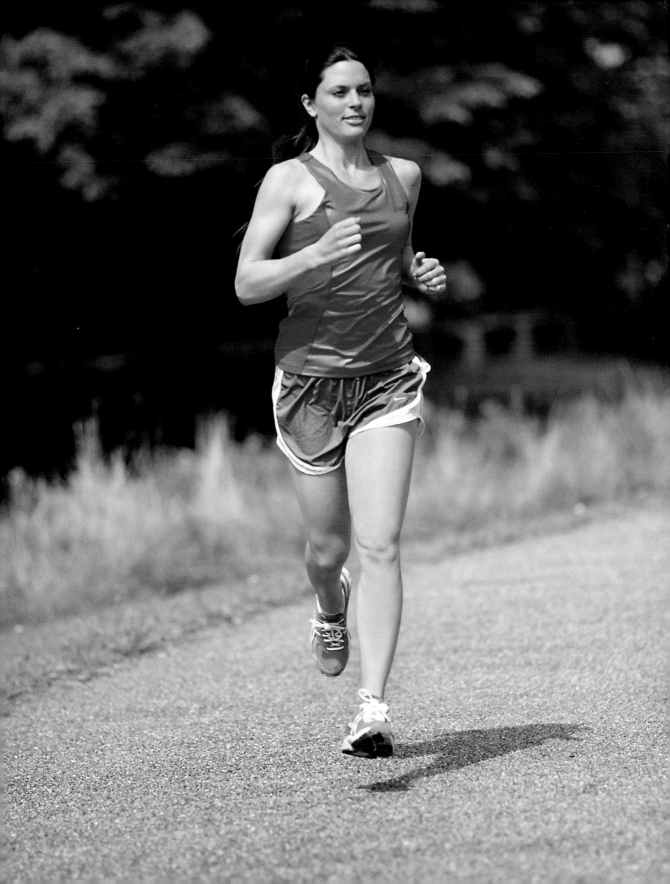

0–20 IN 8 WEEKS

WEEK	1	2	3	
MONDAY	Walk for 2 mins, run for 1 min seven times (21mins)	Walk for 2 mins, run for 2 mins six times (24 mins)	Walk for 2 mins, run for 3 mins six times (30 mins)	
TUESDAY	Rest or cross-train *	Rest or cross-train *	Rest or cross-train *	
WEDNESDAY	Walk for 2 mins, run for 1 min seven times (21mins)	Walk for 2 mins, run for 2 mins six times (24 mins)	Walk for 2 mins, run for 3 mins six times (30 mins)	
THURSDAY	Rest or cross-train *	Rest or cross-train *	Rest or cross-train *	
FRIDAY	Walk for 2 mins, run for 1 min eight times (24 mins)	Walk for 2 mins, run for 2 min seven times (28 mins)	Walk for 1 min, run for 4 mins seven times (35 mins)	
SATURDAY	Rest	Rest	Rest	
SUNDAY	30-min brisk walk	30-min brisk walk	30-min brisk walk to include 3 mins jogging in each 10 mins	

4	5	6	7	8
Walk for 1 min, run for 4 mins five times (25 mins)	Walk for 1 min, run for 5 mins four times (24 mins)	Walk for 1 min, run for 6 mins four times (28 mins)	Walk for 1 min, run for 8 mins three times (27 mins)	Walk for 1 min, run for 10 mins three times (33 mins)
Rest or cross-train *	Rest or cross-train *	Rest or cross-train *	Rest or cross-train *	Rest or cross-train *
Walk for 1 min, run for 4 mins five times (25 mins)	Walk for 1 min, run for 5 mins four times (24 mins)	Walk for 1 min, run for 6 mins four times (28 mins)	Walk for 1 min, run for 8 mins three times (27 mins)	Walk for 1 min, run for 10 mins three times (33 mins)
Rest or cross-train *	Rest or cross-train *	Rest or cross-train *	Rest or cross-train *	Rest or cross-train *
Walk for 1 min, run for 4 mins seven times (35 mins)	Walk for 2 mins, run for 8 mins three times (30 mins)	Walk for 2 mins, run for 10 mins three times (36 mins)	Walk for 1 min, run for 8 mins four times (36 mins)	Walk for 2 mins, run for 12 mins three times (42 mins)
Rest	Rest	Rest	Rest	Rest
30-min brisk walk to include 4 mins jogging in each 10 mins	1.5 mile (2.4km) timed run. Walk where you have to. See p. 31 to rate your progress.	40-min brisk walk to include 5 mins jogging each 10 mins	40-min brisk walk to include 10 mins jogging in each 20 mins	Run for 20 mins

*Cross-train means do an alternative activity. My top choice would be strength and stability exercises – see Chapter 5. Yoga or Pilates would also be great. If you'd prefer to do aerobic activity, pick something that doesn't put too much impact on your joints, such as swimming, cycling or rowing.

These will help to make your muscles, connective tissues (tendons, ligaments, etc.) and bones more fatigue-resistant and, more importantly, injury-resistant. So while you are building your 'aerobic' base (endurance), you are building a musculoskeletal system that can support its demands. You could do strength training on the days marked 'rest or cross-train' (see below) – but if you're struggling to squeeze it in, I'd even go as far as to recommend substituting one of the weekday runs for a strength workout. See Chapter 5 for more about strength and core stability.

Troubleshooting for newbie runners

Don't lose heart if you hit setbacks along the way. Here are some of the most common beginner snags, and what to do about them...

My muscles feel sore

It is normal to feel a little achy and sore after running in the first few weeks. The key is distinguishing between 'good' and 'bad' pain. It's fine to run again if you have generalised soreness, but if you have a specific area of pain in a muscle or joint, follow the steps outlined in Chapter 9 and take a couple of extra rest days. Never run through pain.

I get breathless when I run

Running increases your breathing frequency (your number of breaths per minute) by 300 per cent to get more oxygen into the body for the working muscles to use. So feeling breathless while you run is completely normal. But make sure you're not trying to go too fast – your breathing should not be 'ragged' and out of control, but rhythmic and controlled, even if it's faster than usual. You might find that warming up for a little longer at the start of your session aids the transition into running more comfortably.

I can't fit in four days per week

If you want to run only three times a week, skip the Monday session. Twice a week? Skip Monday and Friday, but expect to progress at a slower rate. Try not to miss the Sunday session – this aims to get you accustomed to being on your feet for longer periods and gets you into the swing of putting aside time for what will become your 'long run'. You don't have to do the sessions on the days stated – but make sure that you spread them evenly throughout the week and don't be tempted to squeeze in extra sessions.

I am not progressing as quickly as the programme says

That doesn't matter one bit. No training programme is written in stone. If you don't feel ready to move up to the next week's schedule, repeat the previous week as many times as necessary. If the sessions feel too easy for you, try moving a week ahead. There isn't a deadline for becoming a runner, so enjoy the journey rather than forcing yourself to progress at an uncomfortable rate.

I got halfway through and I gave up

Well done for getting halfway! Don't see this as a failure; it's simply unfinished business. Try again; but try to pinpoint what caused you to quit. Were you self-conscious about running outside? Try to recruit a friend to go with you, run on a treadmill, or go early when there's no one around. Did you find you just couldn't fit it in? Resolve to stick to three sessions next time and schedule them in your diary like any appointment. Getting to the bottom of what caused you to stop is the key to getting you started again. Check out 'Five ways to make becoming a runner …' on p. 32 for tips to help you next time – find more advice on improving your staying power in Chapter 8.

Measuring your progress

Nothing is more motivating than progress, so it's a great idea to keep tabs on how you are improving as the weeks pass. A caveat: it can take around five to six weeks to see an improvement in fitness (you may feel the benefits sooner) – so don't expect miracles overnight. Bear in mind that how quickly you progress is dependent on many factors, from your age and existing fitness level to how much effort you put in, your diet and lifestyle.

The 1.5 mile (2.4km) timed run scheduled in Week 5 is one measure of how you are doing (see the box below), and you can repeat the test in future months. I also recommend finding other yardsticks of progress; perhaps your running technique has improved, or you're able to extend a little further in your post-run stretch, or you're getting better at judging your pace. That way, if your speed hasn't improved, you've still got other reasons to keep going. And don't start comparing yourself to anyone else – whether it's a friend who started running at the same time as you or your partner who's been a runner for years. No one else has the same physiological (or psychological) make-up as you, so such comparisons are meaningless.

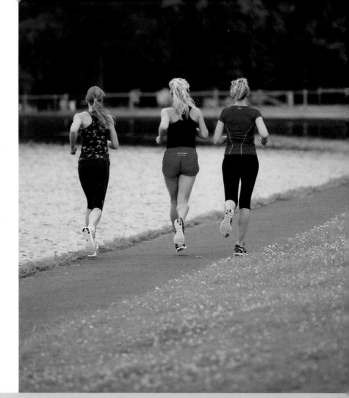

The 1.5 mile run test (in minutes)

The 1.5 mile (2.4km) test involves covering a measured, flat route as quickly as you can. Try to run or jog at a steady pace (in other words, don't sprint for two minutes and then walk the rest). It's a good idea to take someone along, to time you and give encouragement.

Record your time and repeat the test after 8–12 weeks to see how you've improved. You can also compare your time to the 'norm' scores in the table below, but don't get too caught up with this; it's better to compare your own scores as you repeat the test.

Age	Under 30	30-34	35-39	40-44	45-49	50-54	55-60
Excellent	≤10	≤10.30	≤11	≤11.3	≤12	≤12.45	≤13
Very good	10.01–12	10.31–12.30	11.01–13	11.31–13.30	12.01–14.00	12.46–14.55	13.01–15.40
Good	12.01–13	12.31–13.30	13.01–14	13.31–14.30	14.01–15	14.56–16.00	15.41–17.00
Average	13.01–14	13.31–14.30	14.01–15	14.31–15.30	15.01–16	16.01–17.05	17.01–18.10
Room for improvement	≥14.01	≥14.31	≥15.01	≥15.31	≥16.01	≥17.06	≥18.11

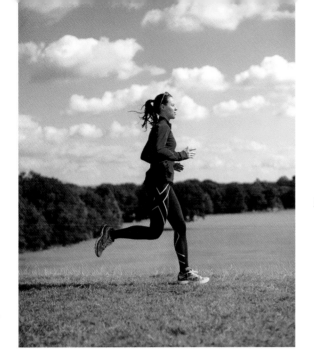

Twenty minutes and beyond

Whether it takes you eight weeks, a fortnight or four months, you will reach the magic 20-minute mark. You'll be able to run without stopping for 20 minutes. So where do you go from there? The next goal is to continue developing your 'aerobic base' – the foundation of your running fitness.

To do this, increase your weekly running time by adding two minutes to each continuous run. And if you haven't done so already, gradually reduce and phase out walking in your walk–run sessions until you are running continuously. Once you reach 30 minutes, add three minutes to each session per week until you can run steadily for 40 minutes. At this point, you'll be ready to start introducing some 'proper' training to your schedule (see Chapter 4).

Five ways to make becoming a runner a happy and successful experience

1. Get some support. Whether it's your partner, your best friend or a local club, make sure you have someone who loves the idea of you being a runner. They don't have to run with you, but being asked how you're getting on, encouraged and motivated is a key factor in making running enjoyable. Compare your partner saying, 'I don't like you going running – it's really dangerous for you to be out on your own,' to 'You're doing brilliantly with this running programme – how far did you get tonight?' I rest my case.

2. Always be prepared. It might sound like the Scout's motto, but, as the saying goes: we don't plan to fail, we fail to plan. Sit down with your diary and plan when you are going to run. Then organise your schedule to fit it in. If you're having a moment of self-doubt, it's harder to ditch the idea if your running shoes are by the front door, your kit is out and the kids are at school. (For more advice on fitting running into your life see pp. 34–37.)

3. Be positive. Don't go out saying, 'Oh-oh, this is going to hurt,' or 'Everyone's laughing at me.' Focus on how you're improving your health, how your body's going to look when you're super-fit, congratulate yourself on making time for yourself. Find a positive about every run – a kestrel soaring overhead; perhaps a passer-by said something nice, or you ran with a friend and had a great catch up.

4. Write it down. I still have my first training diary and I love looking back at how I've progressed over the years. It's also useful for gaining clues on where your natural strengths and weaknesses lie, and it can flag up when you're doing too much or, conversely, jog your memory if you've let things slip! See p. 158 for advice on starting a training diary.

5. Reward yourself. Preferably not with fish and chips on the way home but with some new kit to help your training – or an indulgence, like a massage or pedicure. Your reward doesn't have to be to do with running, but it's nice to connect running and pleasure together in your mind. Nor does it have to be costly; why not take a siesta after your run, or have brunch with your running buddy?

Getting the habit
Make running a part of your life

Finding time for exercise is one of the biggest challenges women face. But with a little forethought and planning, you can make running part of your routine. The beauty of this is that when something is routine, we don't think about it before we do it. We don't weigh up the pros and cons of brushing our teeth each evening – we simply do it.

How do you make running a habit? Figuring out when and where running will fit into your lifestyle is essential. The more disruption it causes, the more likely it is to fall off your 'to-do' list. Try to establish a routine that involves other people. If friends are waiting for you in the park, you're not going to let them down; if you've paid a babysitter so you can go for a run, you're more likely to go.

Being clear about what you want to get out of running is helpful. Your goals don't have to be smashing PBs – they could be increasing your weekly distance, losing weight or finishing a charity race. Once you know where you are going, it's a lot easier to plan your route there.

Goal-setting checklist

- Be specific about your goal – if it's weight loss, how much do you want to lose? If it's to increase your distance, what do you want your mileage to be?
- Is your goal realistic and achievable, while still being challenging? For example, do you really have time to exercise six days a week? Would committing to three or four days be more realistic?
- Set yourself a deadline. When is the 5km charity race? When do you want to have dropped a dress size? Be realistic about your target and work backwards from your deadline when formulating a programme.
- Write your goals down, and record your progress as you work towards them.

Have a plan

Once you've established your goals, creating or following a structured programme to achieve them is really important. That way, each run has a specific purpose, taking you closer to your target. If every run is another plod around the block, it doesn't matter all that much if you miss it. But when each run is an essential piece of the jigsaw, its value is evident. Read more about structuring a training programme and different types of run in Chapter 4 or check out the beginners' programme on p. 28 or the 5km and 10km programmes in Chapter 8.

> Like most non-elite women runners, I have to fit training around other commitments. I only have time to train 'properly' once a week, but I like to cross-train by cycling to work or by going for a swim with the family. I also sneak extra activity into my day by running around the football pitch while I am out walking my dogs, or running up the staircase at work.
>
> Joanne

> *Runs with a purpose, such as picking something up from the shops, give you an extra reason to go, killing two birds with one stone.*
>
> *Libby*

Making it happen

Once you have a goal and a plan, it's easier to fit your running in. If your weekly routine varies, try sitting down every Sunday and planning your runs around the coming week's work and commitments. Otherwise, try to carve out a regular time slot. I often schedule my run after walking the dog – I'm already warmed up and can reach my desired pace more quickly. Here are some other ideas to consider:

Go early

Run before anyone else is up and they start encroaching on your time. It can be a struggle to get up earlier (a cup of tea or coffee is a good kickstart), but research from the Mayo Clinic in the United States suggests that early-bird exercisers are more likely to stick with it than those who exercise later. You'll need to go to bed earlier though. Read more about the pros and cons of running at different times on p. 36.

Run to/from work…

… or part way, depending how far it is. This maximises your time and you'll arrive at work or return home feeling invigorated. Take what you need for the week on Monday and bring the dirty stuff home on Friday. See Chapter 6 for tips on buying a running rucksack.

Break it up

If you can't find the time for a longer run, how about two short runs? Research suggests that the amount of 'afterburn' (calories used after exercise to help restore the body to normal) is higher after two short sessions than after a single run of the same duration.

Make it a date

Whether it's a weekly club session or a run with a friend, a running appointment is easier for you to keep and for your family and friends to get their heads round. If Thursday at 7pm is your regular running slot, then going the next day just isn't a good alternative.

Don't go home

With so many distractions at home – from TV to household chores – it's often easier to extract yourself when you are physically away from home. Perhaps you could run after work, even if it's on the treadmill at a nearby gym. This also offers a good delineation between work and home, enabling you to 'park' work stress.

Do lunch

Could you go running in your lunch hour? Research from Leeds Metropolitan University found that lunchtime exercisers increased productivity in the afternoon. Even 20 minutes on a treadmill can accelerate mental processes and enhance memory storage and retrieval, according to University of Athens research. To save time, take a packed lunch to eat at your desk.

Join a gym

Access to a treadmill, cross-training options and space for strength training can be handy. You'll get somewhere to stash your stuff while you go running and be able to grab a shower. Some offer crèche facilities – invaluable for mums trying to squeeze in a workout.

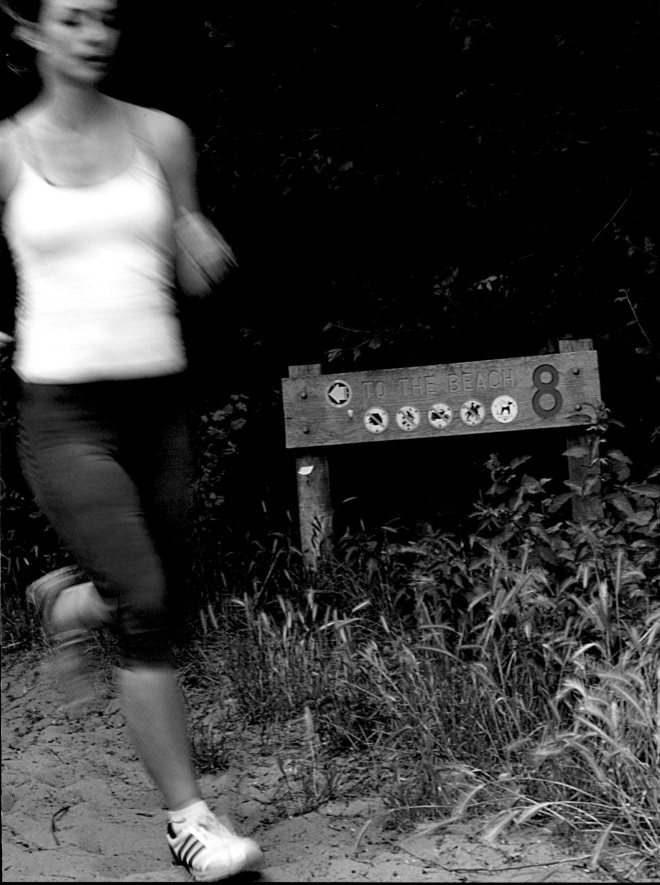

TO THE BEACH 8

The best time to run

Here's how bodily changes throughout the day (circadian rhythms) may affect your running. This knowledge can help you plan your training, but don't get too hung up on timing when you run. It's better to train any time than not at all.

- **On waking** Body temperature is at its lowest and joints are stiffer and drier. Heart rate and oxygen consumption are low. Lung function is at its poorest, so mornings are a bad time for asthmatics to run.
  Points to consider: don't go out when you're still half-asleep – you won't be alert to hazards such as traffic or uneven ground. Allow longer for your warm-up and, if possible, avoid intense sessions, as your chance of injury is higher. Many races take place in the morning, so it's worth practising early-bird runs to prepare.
- **Mid-morning to lunchtime** Adrenaline and cortisol levels are high, so you should feel alert and focused. Body temperature is rising.
  Points to consider: you'll be in a better physiological and psychological state to run than earlier, but you haven't reached your potential physical peak. You might feel more motivated and able to tackle a more challenging session.

- **After lunch** Blood is shunted to the digestive system after eating, making you feel sluggish. There is some evidence that we suffer a 'post-lunch dip' even when we haven't eaten anything.
  Points to consider: allow a couple of hours to digest before running or eat half your lunch before running and the rest afterwards.
- **Early evening** Muscle strength and flexibility, body temperature and anaerobic ability all peak between 4 and 7pm. This is when most athletic records have been set.
  Points to consider: this is the ideal time for a run. Cardiac output is at its highest, improving your endurance, while peak muscle strength will help you to complete tougher speed sessions more easily.
- **Late evening** You may have heard that running close to bedtime will keep you awake, but this isn't true, provided your workout isn't too intense. Researchers found that moderate-intensity late-evening exercise improved the quality of sleep and helped exercisers nod off more quickly.
  Points to consider: a low- to moderate-intensity run is best, followed by a relaxing stretch to cool down.

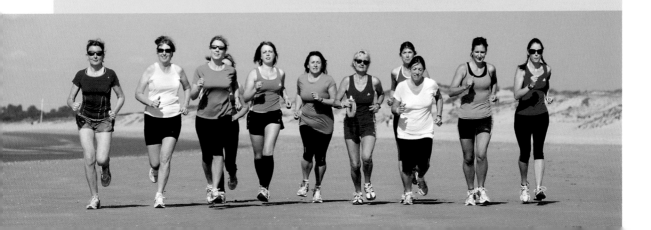

Get organised

Once you know when you are running, get organised to make it happen. Get your kit out the night before early-morning runs (lay it on the radiator on wintry mornings!) and don't organise late-night socialising on the nights before your weekend long runs. If running in the evening, have a mid-afternoon snack so you don't feel too tired.

Be flexible

Contingency plans are the runner's best friend. You may not have time to do your planned session due to other commitments, but could you do a 20-minute jog? If it is torrential rain, could you do your hill session on the treadmill? If your knee is niggling, could you substitute a strength workout? The idea is not to have an 'all-or-nothing' approach. Just because you can't do what you set out to do, it doesn't mean there's no point in doing anything. As my first coach used to say, running once a week is still four times a month more than most people. Some runners like to have a 'fallback' run (such as a 3 mile or 5km no-brainer) that they can do when the planned session isn't doable. While you might feel disappointed that you couldn't stick to the schedule, you'll feel better doing something, rather than nothing.

Make your training varied

Boredom is the enemy! Don't get into a rut by repeating the same sessions week after week. You can vary almost everything about your runs – the pace, the route, the length, the time of day.

Switching between solo runs and runs with others is another way to ring the changes. Training partners not only make running more sociable, they give you another reason for going. Although I love running on my own, I really enjoy my group sessions – and the occasional run with my husband (when I can keep up) and my dog (when he can keep up). See Chapter 8 for more information on running buddies.

Make it a priority

Don't put your needs bottom of the list. Of course you have other commitments and chores, but schedule running as you would any other important appointment. If you adopt a 'wait-and-see-if-I-have-time' approach, you'll never do it. Remind everyone – and yourself – how much happier and energised you'll be after a run.

Have a role model

I have many running heroes: Australian coach Percy Cerutty, for daring to challenge how runners should train back in the 1950s, Paula Radcliffe for her determination and single-mindedness, Roger Bannister for showing us what can be achieved if we set our minds to it and Eddie Izzard, for demonstrating that running is as much about mental strength as physical. It's great to have someone who inspires and motivates you – whether it's someone you know or a running legend.

> "
>
> Run with a buddy or two. I meet up with two friends once a week for a regular half-hour run. Three is a good number, because if you can't make it one week, the other two can still have their run together. On the other hand, more than three and it might be too easy to make excuses.
>
> Elly
>
>

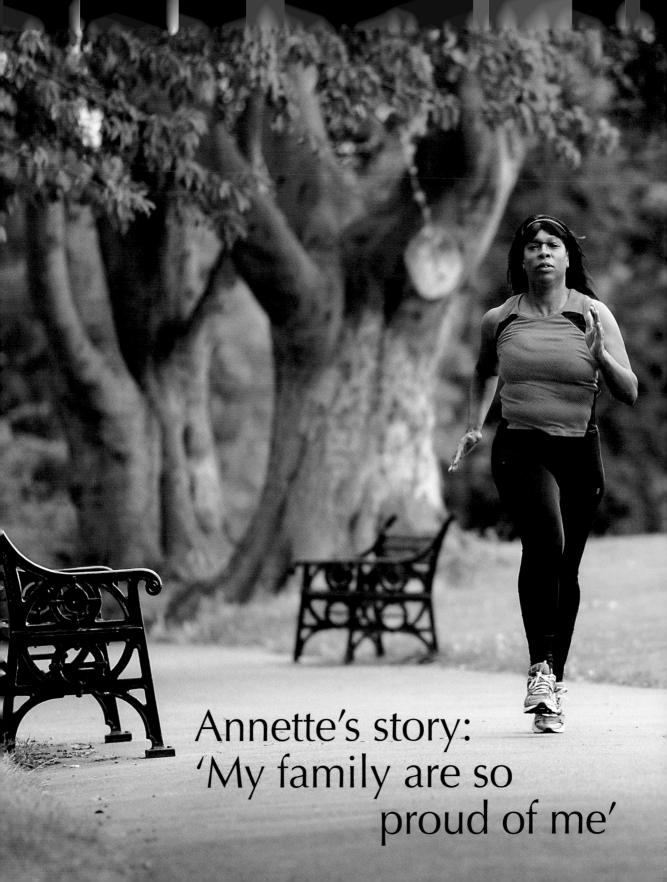

Annette's story:
'My family are so
proud of me'

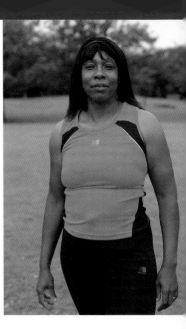

"I will never forget my first run. There I was, 45 years old, jogging along, out of breath and sweating, when I thought I could hear the sound of someone clapping. Then I realised it was my thighs slapping together! That was enough to make me resolve to stick with my exercise plan.

Two and a half years on, I've run a half marathon and set up my own running group, and I can't express how much running has changed my life.

I'd always enjoyed running at school, but in more recent years I'd become completely sedentary and gained a lot of weight. With a high incidence of stroke in my family, my doctor was concerned enough to recommend that I lost some weight and began an exercise programme.

At first I could barely make it round the block, but I persevered. I would run alone, early in the morning; sometimes it was really lonely and hard to motivate myself. Then I joined a women's running group which made the whole experience more fun and social, and really motivated me to carry on. I also set myself the goal of running a 5km event, which gave me something to work towards. When I crossed that finish line, I felt really emotional. I couldn't believe I'd done it. My son and daughter were there watching and they were so proud of me.

I went on to run another 5km race, and then set my sights on the Royal Parks Half Marathon. I was running to raise money for a little boy I knew who had a brain tumour and that was my incentive throughout the training. I was struggling with a hip injury on race day, and probably shouldn't have run, but I was determined to complete the race. I stopped for some assistance from the St John's Ambulance, but when they talked about me dropping out of the race, I just got out of the ambulance and carried on running, even though I was in pain.

To date, I have lost four stone (25kg) and have been given the all-clear by my GP that I am no longer at high risk of having a stroke. I'm delighted to see the effect my running has had on my family too. My achievements have shown my kids that they can set and achieve goals in their own lives. They've said, 'If mum can get up and do all of this, we can too.' My husband, sister, daughter, son and nephew all attend my running group now, and what a great time we are all having getting fit together!

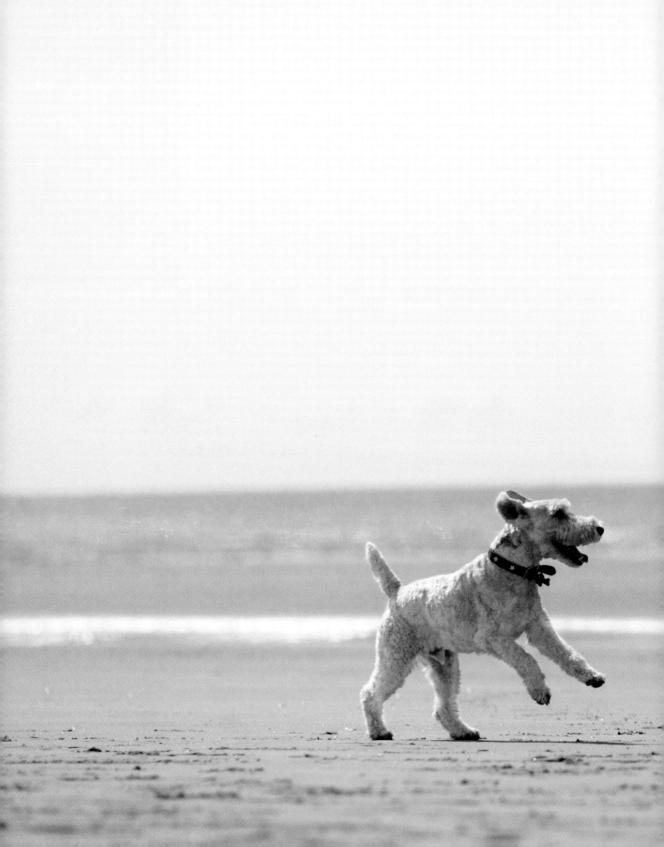

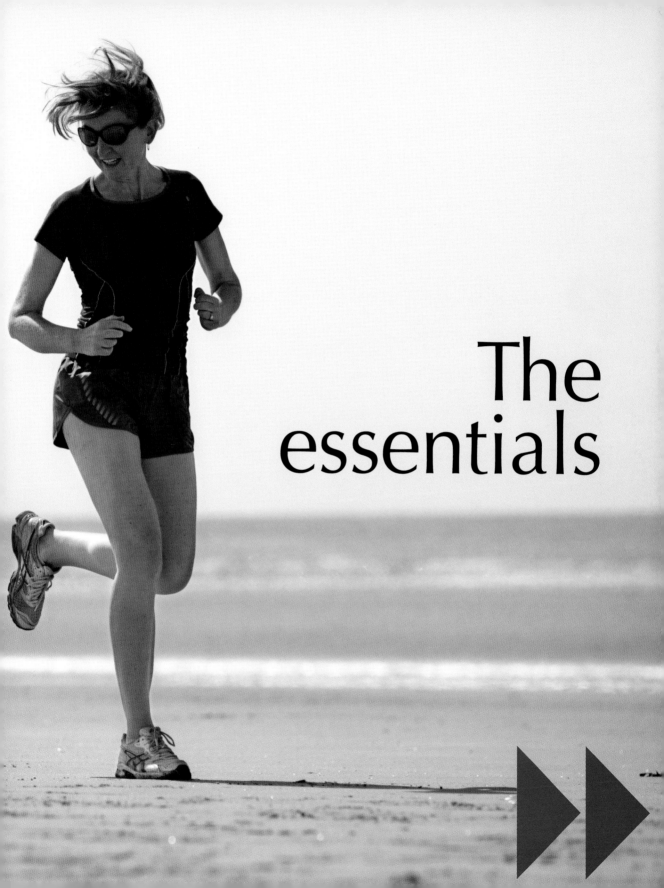

The essentials

Before and after
The warm-up and cool-down

Every run should begin with a warm-up. While the jury is out on many other training practices, the evidence for the value of a warm-up is pretty unequivocal.

Beyond simply warming the body in preparation for exercise, a good warm-up raises heart rate and breathing frequency, increases the release of enzymes for energy production, encourages the blood to release oxygen to the muscles more readily and fires up nerve-to-muscle (neuromuscular) communication, so that muscles contract faster and your stride is more efficient.

Raising body temperature means that muscles become more pliable, so you're less likely to strain them, and the flow of synovial fluid around the joints is increased, lubricating joint surfaces and making movement less stiff.

The upshot is that running feels easier, injury is less likely and performance is enhanced. Not bad for a few minutes of your time! Warming up bridges the gap between your day and your run, allowing a smooth transition and the opportunity to focus your mind. It's as much mental as physical.

How to warm up

Many people jog slowly as a warm-up. This is better than nothing as it raises body temperature, heart rate and breathing frequency – but it doesn't take joints and muscles through their full range of motion or address body parts not directly involved in running. More importantly, it won't 'switch on' neuromuscular pathways. That's where mobility exercises come in (also known as dynamic stretches – I don't use this term because I think it's misleading). Mobility exercises take joints and muscles through their existing comfortable range. These movements are done gently, without yanking or bouncing.

Should you do them before or after a warm-up jog? I like to incorporate them into easy-paced walking and jogging – for example, by walking briskly while raising the knee to hip level on each stride, or slow jogging while taking the arms in large circles. I often add a couple of stationary moves, but make sure I don't remain still for too long to prevent heart rate and breathing from slowing.

Should I stretch?

At one time, stretching (holding a static position which puts a muscle group on stretch) as part of a warm-up was common practice, but over the past decade research has indicated that stretching before exercise is of no benefit, and can be detrimental. If done prior to any form of warming up, like brisk walking, there's a risk of tearing muscles or connective tissues because they are not yet stretchy and elastic. Even after a brief warm-up, there is evidence that static stretching can have a negative effect on performance. In one Japanese study, holding a static stretch for 30 seconds on five muscle groups in the legs reduced power output, whereas mobility exercises increased it. That said, research in 2011 at George Washington University found some support for the argument 'I've always stretched before I run – why should I stop now?' In the study, half the 2,700 participants stretched their quads, hamstrings and calves before they ran, while the other half did not. There was no difference in injury rates between the two groups, but there was a higher propensity to get injured among those who normally did stretch but were instructed not to, and those who didn't normally stretch but were instructed to do so. The study's authors suggest that if it feels good for you to stretch, then do it. My advice is to experiment first with mobility exercises within the warm-up, saving static stretching for after your run.

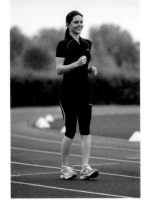
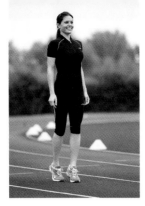
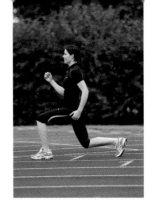
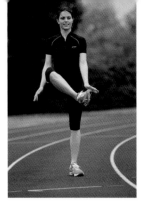

There are two rules to follow when warming up:

- Start slow and easy, gradually increasing your effort and pace.
- Start general, and gradually progress to more running-specific actions.

In an ideal world, you would always warm up. In reality, we are often hard-pressed to fit in a run, and it's warming up (and cooling down) that get neglected. If you don't have time for a full warm-up, start with a fast walk or slow jog and work up to your desired pace only when you feel looser and warmer. If you are running first thing, after a long period sitting down or doing faster runs or races, I strongly recommend making time for a full warm-up, even if it means cutting a few minutes off your run.

Four steps to the perfect warm-up

1. Getting started

Start with some brisk walking and easy, gentle mobility exercises. Focus on freeing up the ankle, knee and hip joints but don't neglect the upper body, especially if you've been at a desk all day. You don't need to do all of the moves; choose a few and vary your choices every time.

- **On the move** (aim to cover 10m or so per move):

▶▶ *Heel walking: take small steps, keeping the balls of the feet off the ground.*

▶▶ *Toe walking: walk forwards with the heels raised, as if wearing high heels.*

▶▶ *High knee marching: walk forwards bringing each knee to hip height while keeping the torso upright.*

▶▶ *Heel flicks: walk/jog forwards bringing the heels towards the bottom without arching the back.*

▶▶ *Walking lunges: walk forwards, stepping into a lunge position on each step.*

▶▶ *Hacky sack: walk forwards, rotating the hip and knee out to the side and touching the foot with the opposite hand.*

- **On the spot** (aim for 8–12 repetitions of each move):

▶▶ *Ankle circles: lift each foot alternately and circle it in both directions.*

▶▶ *Hip circles: stand with feet wider than hip-distance and take your hips in a big circle in both directions.*

▶▶ *Side bends: with feet apart, slide your hand down the side of your leg, keeping hips centred and ensuring you don't lean forwards or back.*

▶▶ *Rolldown: drop your head to your chest, and roll down through your spine, with knees slightly bent, until you reach the ground, allowing the weight of your head and arms to hang down; pause, then roll back up, 'rebuilding' the spinal column, vertebra by vertebra.*

2. Taking it further

Progress to a jog to raise heart rate and body temperature. Again, you can incorporate some mobility moves. As you feel looser, use more vigorous exercises with a greater range of motion.

- **On the move** (aim to cover 20m or so per move):

▶▶ *Sidestepping: step or gallop sideways, keeping your feet pointing directly forwards.*

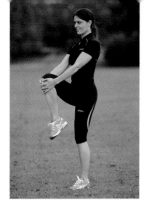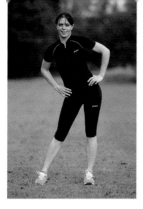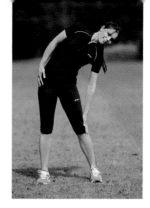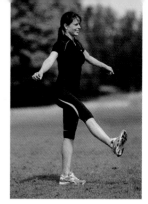

▶▶ *Skipping: skip forwards, lifting the front knee to hip height, and keeping the foot cocked; fully extend the back leg and push off forcefully to get the maximum height per skip. Keep the torso upright and use your arms in a running action.*

▶▶ *High knee jogging: jog forwards bringing each knee to hip height and keeping the torso upright.*

▶▶ *Carioca: step across your right foot with your left foot, then step out with the right foot. Then step behind your right foot with your left foot and step out with the right foot. Once you've got the pattern established, speed up. Travel back leading with the left foot.*

▶▶ *Jogging backwards: just what it says on the tin! Check the area is free from obstacles before you start.*

> I used to prepare for races by jogging and stretching but when I added running at my goal race pace for a few minutes, I found I could get into my stride much more quickly on the gun.
>
> Chris

- **On the spot** (aim for 12–16 of each move):

▶▶ *Side-to-side leg swings: holding a support if you need to and keeping the standing leg straight, swing the other leg out to the side and across the body – keep the movement easy and gentle.*

▶▶ *Forward and back leg swings: keeping the standing leg straight, swing the other leg forwards and backwards; ensure the movement comes from the hip joint and not from the lumbar spine.*

3. Up to speed

Gradually increase your pace or effort to the level required for the session. Steps 1–3 should take somewhere between five and ten minutes and constitute the majority of your warm-up.

4. Know the drill

To prepare for faster running, you may want to shift into your quicker pace by performing a few 'strides': running for 10–20 seconds, focusing on great technique at a swift pace. Or try 'acceleration strides': start at an easy pace and every eight strides speed up a little until you've counted 32 strides. Jog or walk back after each stride and repeat. This is the ideal time to practise technique drills. See pp. 52–53 for more information and some examples.

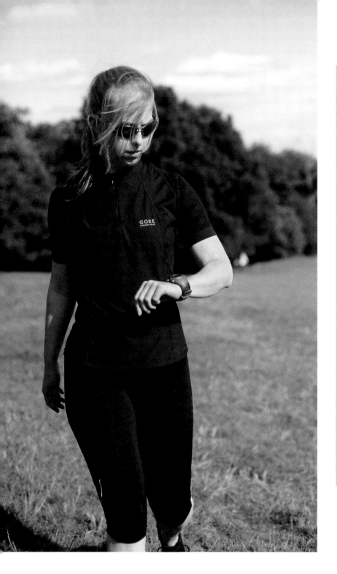

Have a lie-down

Alexander Technique teacher and running coach, Malcolm Balk, recommends a brief lie-down at the end of your run. I've found this very beneficial – a few minutes lying down and focusing on your breathing is a nice way to recover from running and it allows your spine to decompress and tense muscles to let go. Lie face up, with your knees bent and your hands resting on your tummy, elbows out to the side. Keep your eyes open to stop yourself drifting off!

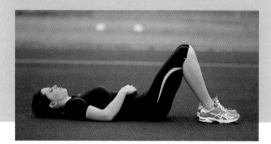

Cooling down

A cool-down is about preparing the body to return to a resting state, allowing those processes that got you ready to run to ease back down. It takes a little time for body temperature to drop, heart rate to slow and breathing to return to normal. If you stop too suddenly, blood still pumping around the body, now no longer needed, may pool in the legs, which can make you feel dizzy or shaky. A few minutes of easy-paced jogging, transitioning to a walk, is all you need to prevent this. The slower your pace and the shorter the run, the less time you need to allow.

Contrary to popular belief, there's no evidence that a cool-down will reduce muscle soreness, but it does ease the return to a resting state and prime you for a post-run stretch (see Chapter 5). An Atlantan study found that performing a cool-down enhanced the exercise experience by allowing you time to take stock of your achievements and enjoy a feeling of accomplishment.

How to run

Why technique matters and how to improve it

You could be forgiven for thinking that there isn't much to running technique – you just put one foot in front of the other, don't you? Well, to an extent, yes. But I am one of a growing number of running coaches who believe that the way you do that – your running technique or 'form' – is very important. There are three reasons for this.

Firstly, efficiency. Running with good technique uses the musculoskeletal system as it was designed to be used, minimising energy wastage, so you have more energy left for the business of travelling forwards. It's estimated that improving technique can boost running economy (your 'miles per gallon' rate) by 2–4 per cent.

Secondly, good technique reduces the likelihood of injury. If there is something a bit 'wrong' with your running stride, you are repeating that mistake approximately 10,000 times for every running hour. It's no surprise that most running-related injuries are 'overuse' ones.

Finally, good technique can make you faster, helping you stay motivated and getting you to the finish line a little bit sooner.

At one time, the belief was that every runner had their own unique running form and attempting to change it, even if it was far from textbook, could create problems rather than solve them. Some experts still believe this, but many others think that just as there's a correct way to swing a golf club or swim breaststroke, there is an optimal technique to running, and as such, that it can be honed and perfected.

I believe that there is an ideal standard, but that in your efforts to achieve it you have to take into account your flexibility and strength (which can be changed), your structural make-up (which can't be changed) and your 'physical history' (you might have broken an ankle in the past, which restricts its range). That doesn't mean you should just accept your limitations – you can work to strengthen weak muscles, just as you can enhance your awareness of your running form and eliminate bad habits. Good technique is not 'all or nothing'. You can run well without perfect form, as a glance at the frontrunners in any race will confirm. And there are degrees of improvement. Even small changes can make a big difference. That's why I like to view running technique as a work in progress.

Is it worth the bother? This depends on what you want to get out of running and how much time and effort you are willing (and able) to put in. At the age of 40, after 21 years of running, I achieved PBs in 10km, 10 mile and half-marathon races by improving my running technique. I wasn't running any more miles in training – I was simply running more efficiently. Working on your form makes good sense. But there's a difference between making a few tweaks to optimise your running style and learning a whole new technique – it is up to you to decide how far to go.

Top form

Here's a brief guide to what your body should be doing in an efficient running posture.

Head Your head weighs 4–5kg so where you hold it affects the stress it places on your joints. One of the most common technique faults I see is looking down at the ground. If you drop your head forwards, its weight throws the spine out of alignment and sends your hips behind you. Don't pull the head back either, as this creates tension in the neck and shoulders. Try to keep your head balanced between the two extremes. Your eyes should be focusing on the route a few metres ahead, not looking at your feet.

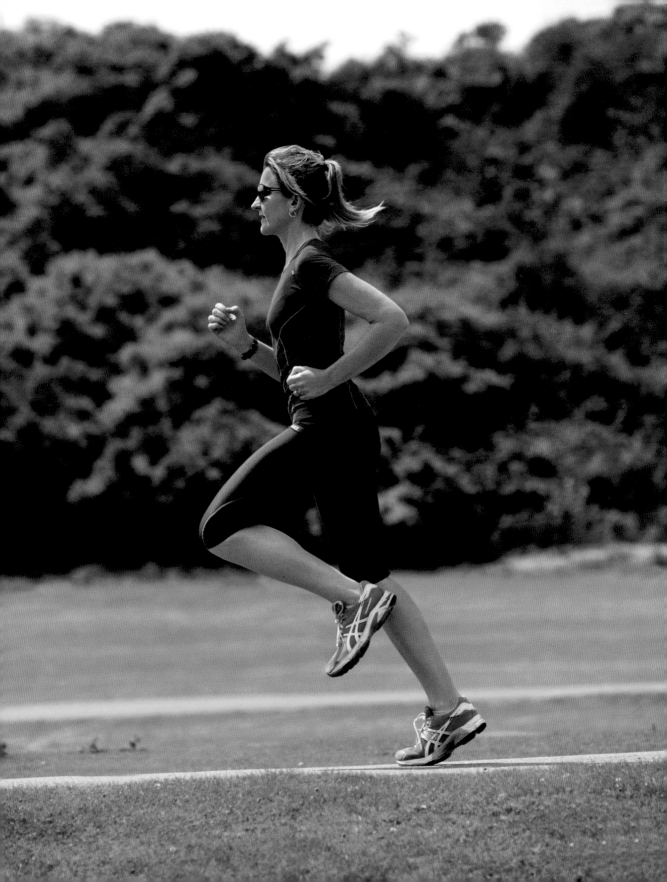

Shoulders Try to keep your shoulders relaxed (imagine your shoulder blades are falling back and down) and your chest open. If you let the shoulders slump forwards, the chest tends to collapse, restricting breathing and raising the likelihood of the arms travelling across your body, which is inefficient.

Arms The arms contribute a lot to the running action, but they often get underused or misused. Not using the arms at all reduces power output, while an overly large range wastes energy. Your pace should dictate your range of movement – the faster you go, the greater the range. The arm action helps to counterbalance the movement of the legs, and, at faster speeds, contributes power to forward momentum. It's important to position the arms correctly, with elbows bent near to 90 degrees and travelling forwards and back, not across the body. Drive back with sufficient force and the arm will spring forwards on its own. The arms can also be used to dictate rhythm: it's impossible to move the arms and legs at conflicting speeds, so moving your arms faster (bending the elbows more helps) can increase your foot turnover (see p. 50).

Hands Clenched fists are not conducive to relaxed running. Nor are hands flopping around like a ragdoll's. 'Relaxed control' is the mantra: imagine you are holding a crisp between each thumb and forefinger – tight enough to keep hold of it, but not so tight that you crush it.

Torso Your torso should be perpendicular to the ground. Visualise lengthening from the belly button to the chest bone, without arching the back, bracing the abdominals or pinning the shoulders back. A slight forward lean is fine, but make sure the lean comes from the feet (so the entire body is inclined forwards), rather than from the hips or waist. To test whether you normally bend at the waist try running with your hands clasped loosely behind you. If you feel as if you are leaning back, it's likely that you have been tipping forwards.

Pelvis A very common error is to 'sit in the hips'. This puts your hips behind rather than beneath you, reducing your power and encouraging a heel strike (see p. 50). Imagine your pelvis as a bucket of water: if it tilts forwards, you spill water out the front; if it tips back, you spill water out the back. Find a central position where you won't spill any and try to maintain this as you run. Maintaining a 'neutral' pelvis requires a certain amount of muscle strength and stability, see Chapter 5. Visualising growing taller with every stride – rising up from the pelvis rather than sinking down into it – can also be helpful.

Legs – Back leg The leg extends behind the body before the knee bends and the heel travels up towards the bottom (how far will depend on your speed and flexibility) to pull through for the next stride. Strong hip extensors (the glutes and hamstrings) and supple hip flexors help to maximise extension power. After extension, bending the knee more deeply enables you to bring the leg through more quickly (it's quicker to move a shorter lever than a longer one).

Front leg Visualise the knee, rather than the foot, leading the stride, and drive it forwards, not upwards. As the leg comes down to land, the shin (which is in front of the knee) should start to pull back so that it lands beneath the body, rather than in front. See pp. 49–51 for more about footstrike.

Ankles and feet Think fast and light. The less you can hear your footstrike, the less impact you are making, and the better it is for your joints. Don't 'push off' your toes as your foot leaves the ground or hold your ankles rigid.

Step by step

The way you run is called your 'gait'. A good running gait is relaxed, fluid and symmetrical with a fast, light footstrike below your centre of gravity. But what do you actually do?

The running gait has three distinct phases – stance, swing and float. While one leg is in the stance phase (foot on the ground), the other is in the swing phase, and then vice versa. The float happens in between, when neither foot is on the ground.

The stance phase begins the moment your foot touches down. In an efficient running stride, the foot lands below, or a little in front of, the body. If you were to place a plumb line along the body, the shoulder, hip and ankle would be aligned, with the torso erect and not bending forwards at the waist.

At the moment of contact, the foot rolls in (pronates) and the arch of the foot flattens, to help absorb the impact. This much-maligned pronation is a normal part of the gait cycle; it's only when the extent of pronation is excessive that it can become problematic because it can cause the shin, knee and hip to roll in too, placing stress on the joints.

The ankle and knee bend at footstrike to help absorb impact forces – the shin and calf muscles work together to stabilise the ankle, while the quads and hamstrings control the knee. The stance leg stores elastic energy (like a stretched rubber band) from the landing within its tendons and connective tissues.

Contrary to popular belief, the first point of contact isn't where the body undergoes the greatest force. That comes a moment later when the ankle, knee and hip extend in preparation for 'toe off'. The elastic energy stored during the stance phase is released to propel the body forwards. The more of this 'free' energy the body can utilise, the less it has to draw on muscular effort. As the foot prepares to take off, the arch stiffens and the foot rolls slightly outwards into a 'supinated' position, giving greater leverage to push off.

While the foot of the stance leg leaves the ground,

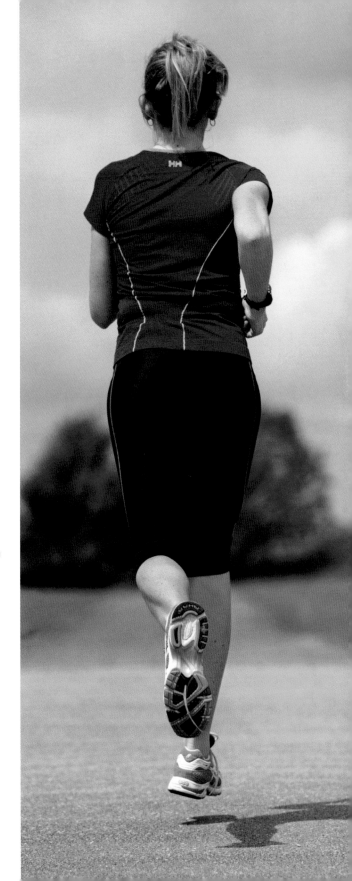

extending behind the body, the swing leg is driving forwards in preparation for landing. For a brief moment, you are airbound in the 'float' phase. Despite the heckler cry of 'knees up', the knee of the swing leg is actually driven forwards not upwards. This leg begins to straighten as you approach touchdown, but the shin and foot start to pull back before contact (like a bull preparing to charge) – this ensures that you don't land on an outstretched straight leg (increasing braking forces) and that you are aligned over your centre of gravity, so you can move quickly into your next stride.

All this happens faster than the eye can see. In an efficient gait cycle, each foot might spend 0.2 seconds on the ground and 0.5 seconds in the air – but a number of things can slow your stride and compromise efficiency.

What goes wrong?

The most common technique fault is 'overstriding' where your foot lands too far ahead of your pelvis (your centre of gravity). When the foot lands in front, it has to stay on the ground longer, 'waiting' for your body to travel over the leg before it can release back off the ground.

"

Don't try to focus on your technique the whole time – it makes you tense and takes the enjoyment out of running. I spend a few minutes at the start of a run working on some aspect of my technique and then I let it go.

Sandra

"

That increases your ground contact time, slowing the gait cycle. You lose that elastic energy stored in your muscles and tendons and have to use more energy to get off the ground. (Try jumping up in the air, landing and pausing for five seconds. Do it a few times. Compare that to jumping consistently without a break. In the second scenario, some energy from the previous landing contributes to the next jump – that's elastic energy.)

When the foot lands in front of you, the leg tends to be straighter, which increases the stress going through the joints, particularly the knee. A recent study found that runners who shorten their stride by 10 per cent reduce the risk of shin injuries by 3–6 per cent. See p. 52 for drills to help avoid overstriding.

Won't landing 'underneath yourself' mean you can't cover as much ground with each stride? Yes, to a degree – but the 'distance' you'd gain from sticking your leg out further is outweighed by the extra time you spend with that foot on the ground (not to mention the increased forces on the joints). In an efficient gait, shorter stride length is compensated for by the speed at which the feet turn over – 'cadence' – and measured in steps per minute. While efficient distance runners usually have a cadence of 180 steps per minute (three strides per second) or higher, less experienced runners often run at a slower rate, yielding a heavier, plodding stride. See p. 53 for how to measure and improve your cadence.

Happier landings

Another common technique problem concerns how – and where – the foot strikes the ground. The long-held belief that some people naturally hit the ground with the ball of the foot first (forefoot or midfoot strikers), whereas others hit the ground heel first (heel strikers), has been strongly challenged in recent years. It is now thought that in an efficient, natural running stride, the foot always lands with the ball of the foot slightly before the heel – it's how we would run if we were barefoot, which is how the body was designed to run.

I agree with this in principle – and I think that

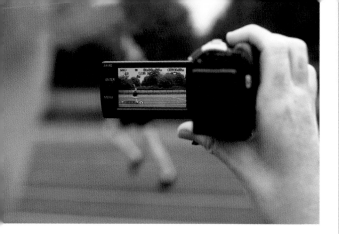

landing with your foot very flexed (so that the heel lands considerably sooner than the rest of the foot) is far from ideal – but there are degrees of heel strike. I'd argue that the position of the foot on initial contact is more important than the part of the foot that hits the ground first. Some elite runners land with a slight heel strike, but the foot still touches down very close to their centre of gravity. Conversely, I've seen runners landing on the balls of their feet who are still extending their legs out in front of them.

If this is getting a little mindboggling, here's an exercise to help: stand up and jump off a chair or step. If you're not able to, just imagine doing so, and ask yourself:

- Which part of your foot lands first?
- Where do your feet land in relation to your body?
- What happens to your knees?

Hopefully, you'll find that the foot lands beneath the body, with the ball slightly before the heel. The knees are bent, to help dissipate some of the impact. The goal in running is to do exactly the same, only with one foot at a time.

I believe that many problems with footstrike stem from regarding running as similar to walking, but faster, when the biomechanics are quite different. Running is more like cycling than walking, with movement happening below the body, not in front of it.

Assessing your form

If you suspect you have serious technique issues, it's a good idea to book a gait analysis with a sports podiatrist

Breathe easy

What's the best way to breathe? The simple answer is which way ever feels easiest and most comfortable. Although some people advocate nasal breathing, research from Liverpool John Moores University found that for 'moderately hard' exercise, the most efficient way of breathing in and out is through the mouth. Similarly, there are proponents of 'belly breathing', where the abdomen expands as you inhale to increase your available lung capacity. I don't recommend this while running as it reduces stability around the pelvis and lower back by removing the 'corset' support of the deep abdominal muscles, which should be lightly engaged as you run. What I do think helps is synchronising your breathing with your footfall in order to get a good rhythm going – breathe in (left foot, right foot), breathe out (left foot, right foot).

or physiotherapist (see Resources, p. 204). A full gait analysis (as opposed to one that takes place in a running shop) usually involves a static assessment, plus walking and running on a treadmill while you are observed from all angles. It isn't necessary for everyone, but it can be helpful in the face of recurring injuries or if you are serious about improving your running form.

You can learn a lot by getting someone to video you running and watching the playback. Get them to film you from the side and back and, ideally, use a camera that enables you to watch the footage in slow motion.

A session with a running coach is another way of getting valuable feedback on your technique. A good coach will be able to suggest appropriate drills, as well as strength or flexibility exercises, to help you remedy any problems.

Technique drills

The following technique drills will help you to improve your footstrike pattern and technique and increase your cadence. Ideally do these at the end of your warm-up or after an easy run.

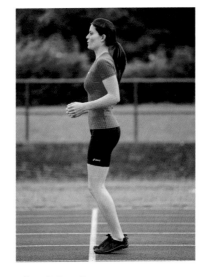

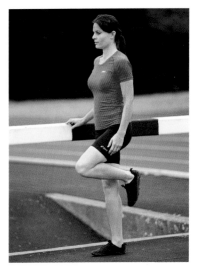

Rules for improving technique

- Focus on one thing at a time – you can't change everything at once.
- Relax and breathe freely.
- After going through a drill, try and put it into practice straight away by running a short distance.
- Remember that any degree of improvement is worthwhile – you don't have to achieve absolute perfection.
- Little and often is best – practise when you are fresh, not fatigued.

Elasticity jumps

Aim: to get the foot landing below your centre of gravity; improves elasticity of lower leg tendons and muscles.

Stand tall with feet below hips, knees and ankles 'soft.' Begin to bounce on the spot, allowing first your heels and then your whole feet to come off the ground. Feel springy but stay low and keep the rate of the bounces very quick (a metronome set to 180 is helpful). Don't 'push off' into the air. Aim for 1–3 x 20–30 seconds.

Leg cycling

Aim: to get a feeling of the leg's 'drawing back' action and strengthen the hamstrings in pulling the foot towards the bottom.

Stand tall and take one foot off the ground. Take the foot through a smooth cycling action, bringing it up under the bottom, driving the knee forward and finally letting the lower leg drop, skimming the ground briefly as the foot passes under the hip. Don't 'dig' the heel in, but land with the ball of the foot first. Aim for 1–3 x 20–30 cycles per side.

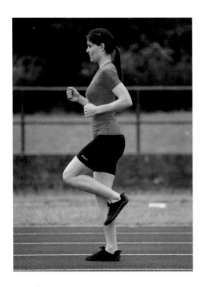

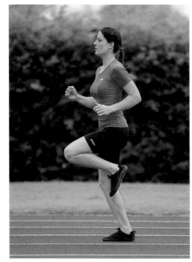

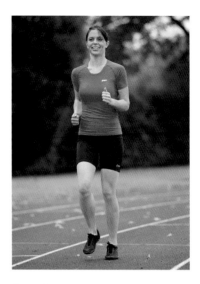

Exchanges

Aim: To help focus on pulling the foot up rather than pushing off; challenges balance.

On the spot, make a 'number 4' shape, with your foot raised, lower leg crossing over the line of your support leg. 'Exchange' to the other side by pulling the support foot off the floor and dropping the other foot to the ground. Don't bend forwards from the waist or hips. As this gets easier, make the exchange more rapidly and try holding the position every third step, with good balance and posture. Aim for 1–3 x 12.

Pick-ups

Aim: to help avoid overstriding and to get the feel of the foot landing beneath your body, rather than out in front; teaches you to get the foot off the ground quickly.

Jog forwards, exaggerating the range of motion of the right leg by bringing the heel up beneath the hip on every stride. Make the movement fast and light. Then repeat the drill on the left leg. Once you've got the hang of it, try alternating from right to left every third stride. Aim for 1–3 x 20 per leg.

Fast feet

Aim: to focus on getting the feet off the ground quickly, using elastic energy, rather than pushing off.

Taking small steps, travel forwards with as quick a cadence as possible, maintaining good posture. Keep the feet cocked (don't point the toes) and use your arms to assist you. Aim for 1–3 x 10m.

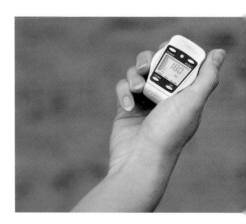

High-cadence jogging

Aim: to improve cadence awareness and help to develop faster leg turnover. (You need a metronome for this one.)

Time yourself for one minute, counting the number of steps you take with one foot during steady-paced running. Multiply this number by two to get your current cadence. Now set the metronome two to four beats faster than that figure and try to match your stride to its beat. Increase by small increments.

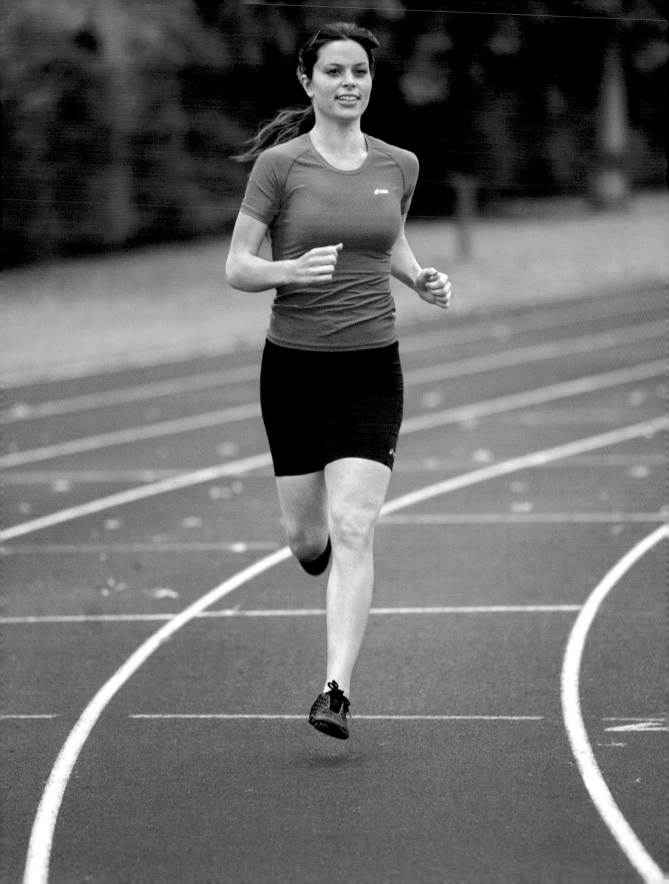

Three more steps to better running

Hours of drill practice isn't the only way to improve your form. Paying attention to the three areas below will also have a beneficial effect.

1. Perfect your posture

Good posture isn't just a matter of standing up straight – it's about being able to maintain optimal body position on the move, even when you are getting tired. This requires strength and core stability, as well as sufficient flexibility in the joints and muscles, which is why I believe that working on these areas is so important for runners.

It's even more relevant for those who spend most of their 'non-running' time sitting down, which shortens the hip flexors and hamstrings, lengthens (and weakens) the glutes and often leaves shoulders hunched and the head jutting forwards from the top of the spine. This is not a posture we want to take into our running! See Chapter 5 to help you to identify any strength and stability shortfalls, and get the lowdown on stretching and flexibility.

2. Raise your awareness

Knowing what constitutes good technique is a prerequisite for running well. But having an awareness of what makes good technique is not the same as actually having good technique! I realised this when I started to use video feedback in my coaching – a rude awakening to my own shortcomings. While external feedback, like video, is useful, it's also important to hone your ability to tune into the feedback your body is giving you. I use 'body scanning' to keep tabs on my posture and technique when I'm running: I might focus on something specific, such as the lightness of my footstrike or I might do a mental 'tour' from head to toe, looking and listening for signs of tension or tightening. This gives me the opportunity to make adjustments to my technique, rather than soldier on with poor form.

For a long time I would get very sore hips when running, but the combination of regular iliotibial band stretching and seriously upping my cadence seems to have eliminated the problem. 'Busy feet' is my motto!

Clare

3. Run relaxed

With so much to think about, the notion of relaxing while you run may sound laughable, but holding unnecessary tension in the body wastes energy and accelerates fatigue. That's why elite sprinters train themselves to stay completely relaxed even when they are running at top speed (check out those floppy jaws in slow-motion television footage).

A warm-up helps to prime your body for a run, dissipating the stress and tension of the day. Body scanning every ten or 15 minutes helps too (the most common sites for harbouring tension are the jaw, the neck and shoulders and the hands). Finally, check you are breathing freely – holding your breath creates tension and anxiety. You could even try smiling!

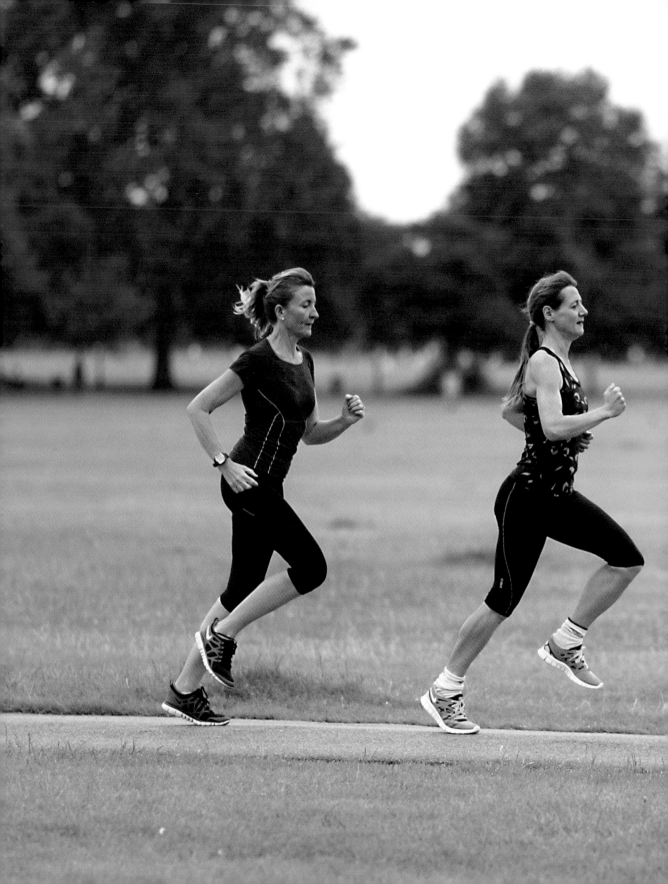

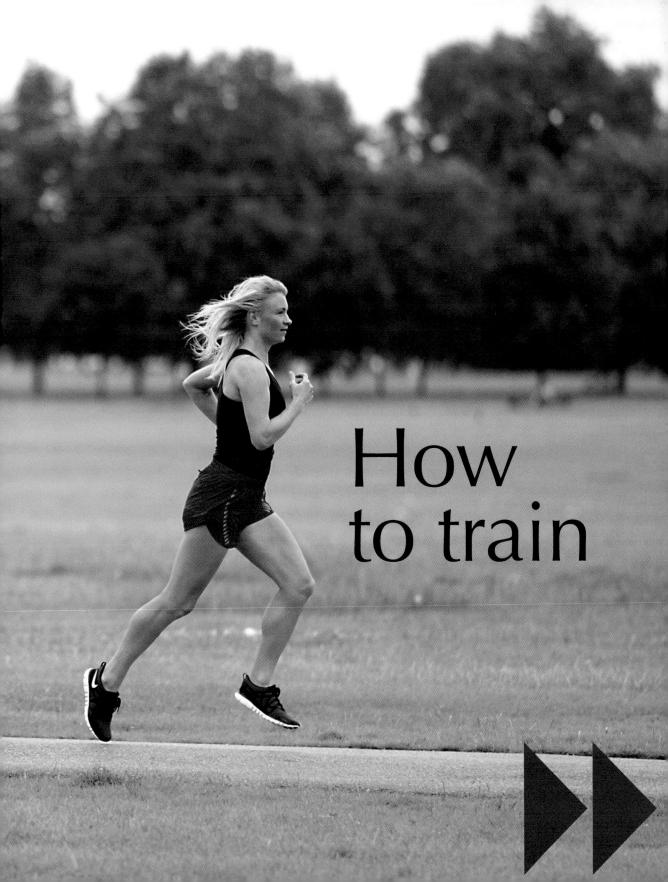

How to train

The rules
How to get fitter, faster

When you take up running, almost any run, regardless of pace or distance, will help you to improve because it challenges your existing fitness. But that's less true as you get fitter. Many runners do the same runs, week after week, with no specific goal in mind. There are two main problems with this, which will limit your improvement. Firstly, if you run at the same speed over the same distance on every run, there is no element of progression. Secondly, there is no variety in the type of challenge being placed upon the body.

If you want to continue to get fitter and faster (even if that doesn't mean going anywhere near a race), there comes a time when you need to structure your training.

Moving the goalposts

Let's imagine your staple run is a 3 mile (5km) steady jog. When you first tackled this, it was probably quite a test for your heart, lungs, joints and muscles, causing them to adapt and strengthen. A few weeks or months on, now that you are fitter, that 5km jog no longer poses a challenge. Without that stimulus, your fitness gains will soon plateau or even decline (it's called 'reversibility').

To continue making gains, you have to slowly but surely increase the stress or 'training load' you place upon the body. Sport scientists call this 'progressive overload'. If you add too little stress, you don't trigger any adaptations, so you don't get fitter – but add too much, and you risk ending up injured or exhausted. The secret is getting the training load right and increasing it at the appropriate rate.

Quality vs quantity

Runners can get very hung up on distance, but progressive overload doesn't have to mean clocking up more miles – you need to strike the right balance of quantity and quality. That brings us to the other problem: lack of variety. Running at different effort levels and on varying terrain yields different physiological and neuromuscular benefits. Run long and slow, and you'll improve your cardiovascular endurance, boost your ability to use fat as fuel and burn lots of calories, as well as strengthening your muscles and connective tissues. But a short, sharp run will improve your VO_2 max (the amount of oxygen your body can extract from the air and utilise in the muscles), raise lactate threshold (see p. 17) and enhance your technique. Throw in some hill climbs and you'll get more muscle fibres working, boosting power and making flat running feel easier, as well as improving running economy. You get the picture!

Get FIT-ter

A good way to remember the options for increasing your training load is the acronym FIT: frequency, intensity and time. These make up your 'training volume'. But which one should you focus on? There's no single factor that is better in terms of progression – a good training programme will play with all three elements will be shaped by what you want to achieve.

'F' stands for frequency: how often are you going to run?

- One of the biggest benefits of running more frequently is that it allows you to inject more variety, as well as increasing your overall volume. Only introduce one additional session at a time, however. Stick with this new weekly total for a few weeks before considering adding another extra session.

'I' stands for intensity: how hard are you going to run?

- Increasing the intensity of some of your running is of great benefit if you want to improve your speed over a given distance, but wait until you can run at a steady pace for 30–40 minutes before introducing tougher sessions. Bear in mind using hills or more demanding terrain can raise intensity without increasing pace.

'T' stands for time: how long or far are you going to run for?

- This is the key variable for beginners to focus on. Increased duration should always precede increased intensity. Adding minutes or miles to your runs is a great way of raising your training volume and building up to longer races like half marathons and marathons.

Striking a balance

When you want to increase your training load, pick one element at a time. Don't try to increase the number of times you run, your pace and distance all at once. That's not progressive. Bear in mind that there's a pay-off between intensity and time – the harder you run, the shorter the session (or it could be broken down into short bouts of effort, as in 'interval training', see p. 64).

A common rule of thumb is to increase weekly mileage or minutes by no more than 10 per cent at a time. This works fine when your mileage is low, but it can ramp things up rather quickly if you are clocking up 25 miles a week or more. A more conservative option is to increase your volume by the number of sessions you run per week in miles every third week. If you run four times a week, you would increase your weekly mileage by four miles every third week, for example.

Rest and recovery

Whichever method you choose, you can't keep on increasing your weekly mileage indefinitely. Those physiological and biomechanical adaptations that occur as a result of progressive overload take place when you are at rest (primarily during sleep), not while you're out running. That is why it's so important to build recovery into your training. One of the best ways of doing this is by following the 'hard–easy rule'. This means structuring your training so that you don't do two hard sessions in a row; it will lower your chances of getting injured and ensure you don't end every week feeling exhausted. See the programme builder on p. 72.

I also recommend taking recovery weeks occasionally, where you scale mileage and intensity right down. Try reducing your training volume every three to five weeks, depending on your experience, goals and how you are feeling. This will keep you physically and mentally fresher.

Be specific

Just as psychologists tell us that our goals need to be specific ('I want to finish a 5km without walking', as opposed to 'I want to get fit', which is too vague), sport scientists talk about 'specificity' in terms of training.

This means that if you want to swim the Channel, you should practise your front crawl; if you want to cycle from Land's End to John o'Groats, get on your bike.

But specificity applies within a sport too. If you want to run a fast road 10km, your training will be very different from training for a hilly cross-country event. That's because the adaptations from training are very specific to that type of training. The perfect example? A group of orienteers (runners who have to navigate cross country to reach specific points) and a group of track runners with equal levels of fitness were assessed running on rough terrain with steep hills. The orienteers used less energy to cover the terrain because they'd tackled this sort of ground almost every day in their training, whereas the track runners stuck to the roads and athletics track. Although both groups were accomplished runners, the exact fitness gains they had achieved were related directly to their mode of training.

Be consistent

Unfortunately we can't 'store' fitness. If you've had a bit of a lull in your training, don't assume that you are still as fit as you were a few weeks or months ago and push yourself too hard. This is particularly true for new runners. Researchers have found that newbie exercisers aren't able to hold on to their fitness for as long as more experienced athletes when they take a break. One study found new exercisers who had trained consistently for eight weeks lost all their aerobic fitness gains after an eight-week break from exercise. If your training has been inconsistent, don't make the mistake of cramming in extra sessions or skipping ahead in the schedule to 'catch up'. Ease yourself back into the swing with a few easy days, and gradually progress from there.

Tailoring your training

To know what type of training you should focus on, you need to have a goal. Training doesn't have to be all about the end result; even as a competitive runner I know that the joy of running isn't just about the finish, but is also about the process of getting there. But knowing that each run is bringing you closer to your goal can add richness to your running. Working towards a goal uses your training time most efficiently and helps you to stay motivated (it's a lot easier to skip 'another run' than to miss your weekly hill session).

In the next section, you can find out about the benefits of different types of runs and their purpose. Coupled with your goal, this should help you to determine what should be in your programme. By following the programme builder on p. 72, you'll be able to construct your own training schedule.

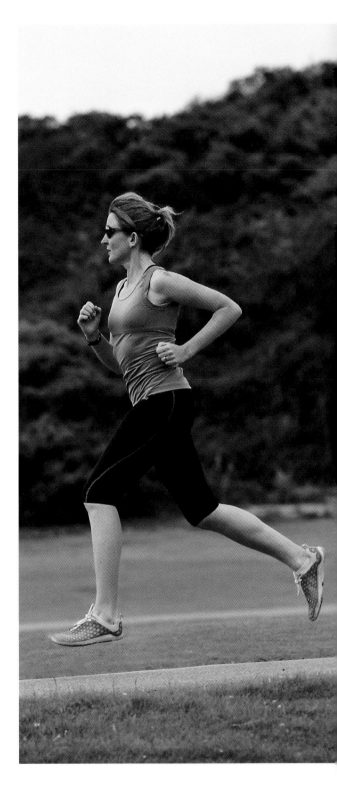

Your training menu
The lowdown on different types of run

There are many ways to run: slow, steady, long and easy, short and sharp, up or down hills, around a track or along a forest trail. Each type has its own unique benefits, and whether it has a place in your programme is dependent on your goals and experience. Read on to find out which are the key sessions for you.

Steady runs

Steady-state runs or 'steady runs' are what most of us instinctively do – putting in the miles at a comfortable pace well below our maximum capability. Steady running isn't so challenging that it leaves you fatigued, so you can do more of it, helping to build your overall volume of training. It improves cardiovascular fitness, burns calories and helps your muscles, tendons and other connective tissues to adapt to the forces of running, reducing injury risk.

The key thing about a steady run is that the pace feels comfortable. You should be able to hold a conversation as you run, albeit a slightly breathless one. (For more about monitoring your effort level see p. 68.)

If you are new to running, all your runs should be steady or easy runs. Only when you've been running consistently for a few weeks and can go continuously for 30–40 minutes should you start stepping outside the steady run 'comfort zone'.

Easy/recovery runs

Easy runs or 'recovery' runs should be slower than steady runs. Runners often do their easy runs too hard, and their hard runs too easy, so training is all of a similar intensity. Far more benefit can be gained from having a mix of easy, moderate and hard runs.

The main purpose of a recovery run is to add some mileage without too much overload – the pace needs to be pretty effortless and the runs shouldn't be too long. Otherwise, rather than assisting with recovery and adaptation, they'll create additional stress. There is some evidence that a gentle recovery run can hasten recovery more than complete rest, so it's wise to schedule them following tougher runs.

Long runs

You might think that long runs are only for those gearing up for marathons, but every runner can benefit from a regular longer run.

> "
> My latest thing is going for a long run/walk. I run as much as I can, but walk when I feel like it. This has enabled me to be out in the countryside for three hours or so, enjoying the sun and scenery and feeling wonderfully exhausted afterwards. It's allowed me to really test my running and extend the time on my feet without ending up injured.
> Elizabeth
> "

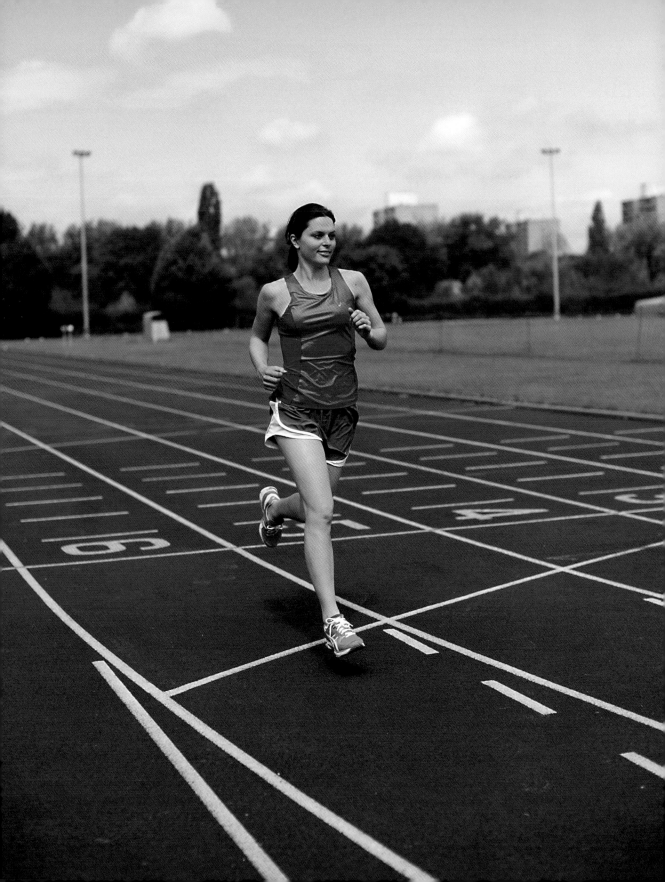

The benefits of long runs are the same as for steady runs, but multiplied, due to the increased duration. You don't have to do a long run every week – once a fortnight is plenty if you're not marathon training – and the term 'long' is relative. To determine your starting point, I recommend adding ten minutes to your current longest run. Do not increase the distance of this run by more than either ten

---

Walk–run

Mixing walking and running is how most of us start running, but that doesn't mean it's not a strategy to adopt later on in your running career.

Walk–run proponents believe combining the two activities can help you keep going for longer and improve race times because it gives you an in-built element of recovery – physically and psychologically. It works particularly well off-road where steep climbs, slippery descents and gates naturally slow you down, but it can easily be built into road running. Perhaps the best place is within your long run, where it enables you to run for longer without over-stressing your body. It also makes you less likely to dread the session.

Start by walking for two minutes after every eight minutes of running or for one minute after every nine (each time your watch hits a round number you need to begin running again) or, if you have a GPS device, you could walk for one to two minutes after every kilometre or mile. This is a golden opportunity to perform a body scan (see p. 55) to spot any niggles.

Unless you are still progressing towards continuous running, don't walk–run every session or you may find it hard to master continuous running.

---

minutes or one mile at a time. Adding some walk breaks (see 'Walk–run') to this longer session can extend your 'time on feet' without overdoing things.

High-intensity training

Long runs, steady runs and easy runs all address the 'T' of the FIT acronym. What about the 'I'? The following sessions will increase the intensity of your training in some way. Don't go overboard – even elite distance runners, who might log 200km plus per week, only do a small number of these sessions. The majority will be easy and steady runs, the 'bread and butter'.

If you are running three times a week or fewer, one high-intensity session is enough. I recommend starting with fartlek (see p. 64) or lactate threshold training (below). If you run four or more times a week, then you could aim for two hard sessions. If your long run exceeds two hours, I recommend counting it as one of them, because the duration becomes the challenge.

Lactate threshold training

Lactate threshold (LT) (see p. 17) is one of the key attributes of a fit runner. The LT is the point when lactic acid in the muscles increases sharply because it cannot be cleared as quickly as it is produced. Training at an intensity around the LT is the best way to improve your threshold, so you can sustain your pace without contending with the negatives of crossing the LT.

What's the right effort level? LT tends to equate to around 85 per cent of your maximum heart rate – or the speed you could maintain in race conditions for up to an hour (this could be your 10km pace, or slightly slower). It's often described as a 'comfortably hard' pace or 'controlled discomfort' but it's not, as people mistakenly believe, an all-out speed session. I use threshold training as the introduction to faster work for newbies who are ready to progress. It's also the key speed session to improve pace in events lasting 30 minutes or longer – up to a marathon.

There are two ways to do threshold training. The standard is to run for 15–45 minutes at a sustained pace (after a warm-up, you maintain your threshold pace or effort level for the duration of the run). This is often called a tempo run. If that sounds daunting, or if you think your session might be pretty short if you have to work continuously, then try threshold intervals. Here, you work at the same pace, but break the session into intervals (no shorter than five minutes, no longer than 15 minutes), divided by short rests. Take one minute recovery for every five minutes of running. This might enable you to do more overall than one sustained effort. For example, four repetitions of five minutes with one-minute recovery jogs (20 minutes at threshold pace) compared to 15 minutes in a single effort – an extra five minutes!

Interval training

Lactate threshold training teaches your body to get comfortable working at a higher proportion of its maximum aerobic capacity. But interval training is geared towards improving the maximum capacity itself – VO_2 max. The higher your VO_2 max, the faster you can run while maintaining aerobic energy production. To train VO_2 max most effectively you need to run at, or close to, the pace that elicits your maximum (remember, VO_2 max is a physiological measurement, not a pace). If you've already done a 5km, the pace you are aiming for is likely to be equal to or slightly faster than what you achieved, on average, over that distance.

Thankfully, you only need to work in short bouts to reap the VO_2-max-boosting benefits of interval training and you get nice long rests in between (that's why it's called 'interval' training). For each minute of effort, allow 30–60 seconds of recovery – the efforts should each last between one and five minutes.

While VO_2 max training is useful for all runners, it's of most benefit to people training for shorter distances, i.e. 5- and 10km races. If you are training for longer distances, it's the 'icing on the cake'. And it's not for beginners.

Speed work

In true speed work, you are no longer working aerobically, because the pace is too fast to supply sufficient oxygen. Your body has to rely on 'anaerobic' (without oxygen) energy production. Whereas easier-paced running relies mainly on 'slow-twitch' fibres in the muscles (those associated with prolonged, submaximal contractions), maximal-paced running calls on 'fast-twitch' fibres too (the ones designed for short bursts of effort). This enhances muscle strength and power. It also improves technique, which should benefit more leisurely paced runs, and give you a 'kick' for that sprint to the finish.

The rule should be 'little and not too often' for speed work. It could be incorporated into another session by adding some fast 'strides' at the end, when your muscles are warm and pliable, or a standalone session of short reps of a specific distance, like 200m, or time, such as 20–30 seconds. Allow yourself plenty of recovery between each rep – two to three times as long as the length of the effort.

Fartlek

Fartlek is a Swedish word meaning 'speed play', and playing with speed is exactly what this is. There's no set schedule, but the idea is to mix hard running with easy jogging, usually on varied terrain. The intensity can be dictated by the terrain – steam up a hill and then jog until you catch your breath, or sprint between every third lamp post – or by your stopwatch.

Fartlek can be a great way to introduce beyond-the-comfort-zone running, as it isn't too structured. But it can be a bit vague for beginners, who aren't sure how many efforts to put in or how fast to go. Plan your session in advance in terms of how many efforts to do and at what pace, and ensure you temper hard bouts with plenty of recovery time.

Hills

Hills are a great way of increasing cardiovascular effort, while building muscular strength in the legs – a Greek study found that 20 per cent more muscle fibres were activated running uphill compared to flat ground. If you are a new runner, try to schedule the hills early in a run before you get tired, when technique is more likely to be compromised.

While I'm a big fan of using hills to increase intensity and improve fitness, it's important that you know what 'type' of hill session you are doing as you would know the purpose of any other session. You could incorporate hills into a fartlek run to add intensity, or into your long run to replicate a forthcoming hilly race. Or you can use hills to work on your lactate threshold or VO_2 max. There are two main types of hill training:

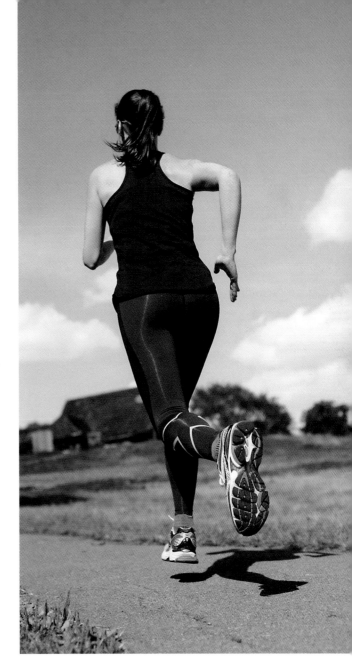

- **Hill reps** In a traditional hill reps session, you run up the hill fast and jog/walk back down to recover. This is a great way to work on your VO_2 max. Look for a hill that will take you between 45 seconds and three minutes to climb, and don't pick one of Everest-type gradient. On a treadmill, try a gradient of 4–6 per cent. Don't time your recoveries – simply take as long as you need to get back to the bottom.

- **Continuous hills** In a continuous hills session (sometimes called Kenyan hills) you run up and down the hill at your lactate threshold effort level (there's no jog down or rest at the bottom) for a given duration or number of reps. The uphill provides an additional cardiovascular challenge and builds leg strength, while the downhill is good for increasing leg turnover. A study in the *Journal of Strength and Conditioning Research* found that runners who trained up and down hills increased cadence and speed more than just running uphill or on the flat. Aim to run at the same effort level you'd achieve running at threshold pace on the flat – the pace itself will be a little slower. I opt for shorter hills, so there are more ups and downs, rather than one or two long climbs and descents; and I avoid hills that are too steep, which might negatively affect technique. Use a more generous 'effort-to-recovery ratio' than on flat ground to account for the added challenge of the hill – one minute recovery for every four minutes of effort.

Rules for high-intensity training

- Warm up for at least ten minutes and include some mobility exercises.
- Pace yourself. Just because hard or fast is good, it doesn't mean harder or faster is better. Try to stick to the effort levels or pace guidelines given for the different types of sessions. See 'Monitoring your effort level' below.
- The key to a good interval, hill or speed session is for all your repetitions to take roughly the same time or to get slightly faster. If you cover 1km in your first effort, and only manage 0.8km on the remainder, you went too fast.
- Always schedule a high-intensity session between two easier ones to comply with the hard–easy rule (see p.59).

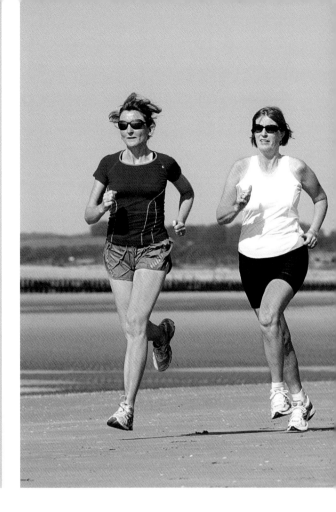

Race pace training

Race pace training isn't about stimulating a specific physiological variable or aspect of fitness, unlike other sessions. Increasingly, coaches are realising the importance of practising 'goal race pace' – the specific pace at which you want to run in your event. If, for example, you want to run 5km in 35 minutes, that equals seven minutes per km. Doing some runs – or bouts within runs – at this pace will help get your body accustomed to how it feels, standing you in good stead on race day.

One area where this has been particularly beneficial for me is in marathon training. Incorporating bouts of running at my goal race pace during my long runs has helped me to 'lock on' to that pace and get comfortable with it. I simulate race conditions by putting the miles at race pace

towards the end of the long run, when I'm getting tired and have to work really hard to sustain the goal pace. This strategy would be useful for shorter races too.

Monitoring your effort level

All the runs outlined above require different effort levels – from almost effortless to flat out. But how do you know whether you are working hard (or easy) enough? Many runners monitor either their heart rate or their running pace to check they are working at the appropriate level for that session. These require mastery of the appropriate gadget (see Chapter 6) and knowing what pace or heart rate is required by the run. For technophobes there are a couple of simpler ways of monitoring effort level.

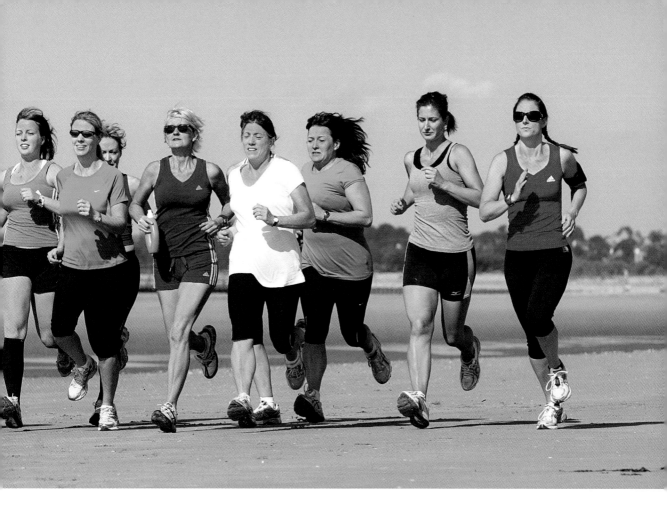

Let's talk

One method is the 'talk test' – how much conversation you can make during a session. At threshold pace, you should only be able to utter short phrases, while at steady-run pace you should be able to hold a conversation. The other method is the 'rate of perceived exertion' (RPE), which describes how hard you feel you are working. It might sound a little unscientific, but research from the University of Exeter found that our built-in ability to assess our effort is surprisingly accurate. When volunteers were asked to 'rate' how hard they were working on a numerical scale, their estimates correlated closely with how hard they were actually working as measured by their heart rate and oxygen uptake. The benefit of RPE is that it is truly individual. If you are on a steady run with a friend, you might rate the pace as 'extremely hard' while they describe it as 'easy'. This indicates that you should slow down, in order to reap the benefits of a steady run. As RPE isn't related to a physiological reading or a specific pace, it also takes into account that you might be feeling a bit low on energy on a particular day.

I have devised an RPE scale of one to five, which I use with clients who don't appreciate scientific jargon. The table over the page indicates how each effort level relates to the talk test, heart rate and pace. Newer runners should stick to the lower end of each range in terms of heart rate. The pace guide is only relevant if you have completed a few races, because training pace is based on your speed in races of varying distance.

How hard am I working?

RPE level 1: effortless pace
Talk test: could chat nineteen to the dozen all day.
Heart rate: 65–74 per cent of max heart rate (see below) or even lower, if necessary.
Pace-per-mile guide: one to two minutes slower than your threshold pace (level 3).
Uses: use on easy runs and the 'recovery' sections of your interval training, hills or fartlek; could be used for long runs, especially when trying to up your distance.

RPE level 2: steady pace
Talk test: could hold a comfortable but breathless conversation.
Heart rate: 75–81 per cent of your max heart rate.
Pace-per-mile guide: half marathon to marathon pace.
Uses: use on steady runs and some long runs.

RPE level 3: challenging pace
Talk test: could eke out short phrases in conversation.
Heart rate: 82–90 per cent of your max heart rate.
Pace-per-mile guide: 10km pace or 10–20 seconds per mile slower.

Uses: use on threshold intervals, tempo runs and continuous hills.

RPE level 4: tough pace
Talk test: one-word answers only.
Heart rate: 91–99 per cent of your max heart rate.
Pace-per-mile guide: 5km race pace or a few seconds per mile quicker.
Uses: use for VO_2 max interval training, hill reps and 5km race-pace training.

RPE level 5: maximal pace
Talk test: no conversation.
Heart rate: equates to 100 per cent of your max heart rate.
Pace-per-mile guide: As hard as you can for the required duration.
Uses: use for speed work.

Working out your heart rate

If you monitor your heart rate, you'll need to know what your maximum heart rate is to determine any given percentage of it. You can have your true maximum heart rate measured in a maximal exercise test in a physiology laboratory, but this isn't really necessary unless you are very serious about your running (see Resources, p. 204 for further details).

The simpler option is to use the 220-minus-age formula. This is a very broad approximation of heart rate – real values can be as much as ten beats out – but it's an acceptable guideline. Subtract your age from 220 to get an estimated maximum heart-rate value. For example, if you are 40 years old: 220 - 40 = 180. Then work out the heart rate corresponding to 65 per cent or 75 per cent of that.

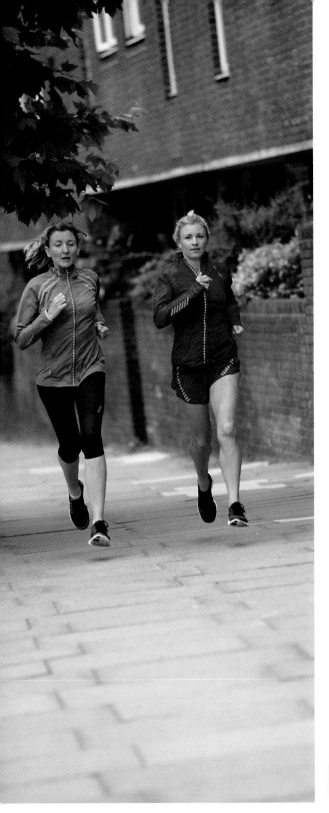

Heart-rate reserve

For a more accurate guideline for how hard you should be working in different sessions, you can work out your 'heart-rate reserve', using the Karvonen formula. This takes into account your resting heart rate (a strong indicator of your fitness), as well as your age-predicted maximum, so is a more fine-tuned method.

First, use the 220-age formula opposite to work out your maximum heart rate (MHR). To find your resting heart rate (RHR), place two fingers on the thumb side of your opposite wrist until you detect the pulse. Time how many beats you feel in one minute. For best results, do this first thing in the morning, before you have risen or had any caffeine. Now, to find out what your heart rate would be if you were working at, say, 75 per cent of your maximum, use the following formula:

75 per cent = (MHR - RHR) x 75 per cent + RHR

Example: you are 40 years old. Your resting heart rate is 60bpm. Age-determined MHR = 180.

75 per cent = (180 - 60) x 75 per cent + RHR

75 per cent = 120 x 75 per cent = 90 + 60

75 per cent = 150bpm

> "
>
> I used to do all my runs at the same speed, but by introducing speedwork and tempo runs, I have upped my overall pace considerably. I have been surprised how much I enjoy pushing myself on the faster runs too.
>
> Jennifer
>
> "

Building a programme
How to make running work for you

As a runner, I'm often asked 'Do you run every day?' or 'How many miles do you run?' The answers, of course, depend on what I am training for, as I don't follow the same schedule when I'm preparing for a marathon as I do when I'm gearing up for a 5km. And the same should go for you.

If you only want to run for fun and general fitness you might question whether you need to structure your training at all. My response would be yes. As well as paving the way for PBs, following a planned programme ensures balance and consistency in your training, which reduces the risk of injury or exhaustion. It also introduces variety and challenge, so maintaining interest.

The principles underpinning successful training and the purposes of different types of run are outlined on pp. 58–69. This section will help you put it all into practice and to construct your own effective training programme, whatever your goals.

Seven steps to creating a schedule

- **Step 1** Determine your goal and the time frame within which you want to achieve it. (See Chapter 2 for information on goal setting.) If it's a race, work backwards from race day to the present: how long have you got? This helps you work out your priorities.
- **Step 2** Assess where you are now. If, for example, you have a weight loss goal, you can use the scales (or a body fat percentage) as a marker of your starting point. If your goal is to run 10km, how far can you currently run? This helps you to check that your goal is realistic and achievable.

- **Step 3** Decide how much time you can commit to attaining your goal. Be realistic – there's no point saying you'll run seven days a week when the demands of family, work and running a home simply won't allow it.
- **Step 4** Decide what your most important focus is going to be in training. Is it going to be threshold training to raise your pace for your next 10km? Or hitting the hills to prepare for a trail event? (To recap on the purpose of different types of session, see pp. 61–66.) Your training focus can change as you progress; for example, once you are comfortable doing a weekly threshold session, you might consider switching to hills or interval training to further develop your speed and strength.
- **Step 5** Based on the outcome of Step 4, identify what will be the most important session of the week. This could be your long run or it could be a faster session or hill workout, depending on your goal. Schedule this session on the day it's most likely to get done (so even if everything else falls by the wayside, you will still get to tick this session off).
- **Step 6** Now schedule two easy days around this key session. An easy day could mean an easy or steady run, a cross-training activity or no activity at all. I certainly recommend having at least one non-running day per week, even if you do a different activity.
- **Step 7** Now pick your next-most important session for that week, as in Step 5, and again, schedule it between two easy days. Repeat the process until you've run out of days. Simple!

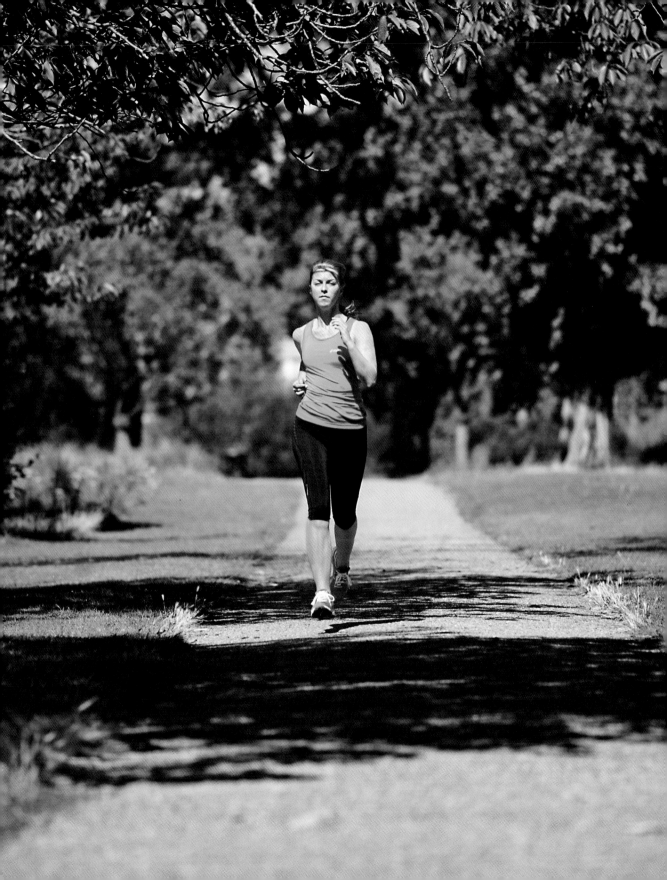

THE PROGRAMME BUILDER: an example

EASY RUN	MONDAY	REST
STEADY RUN	TUESDAY	THRESHOLD
	WEDNESDAY	EASY PLUS SUPPORTIVE TRAINING
REST	THURSDAY	STEADY
CROSS-TRAIN	FRIDAY	FARTLEK
SUPPORTIVE TRAINING	SATURDAY	EASY/CROSS-TRAIN
	SUNDAY	LONG RUN (EASY)
THRESHOLD	MONDAY	REST
VO2 MAX INTERVALS	TUESDAY	THRESHOLD
	WEDNESDAY	STEADY PLUS SUPPORTIVE TRAINING
FARTLEK	THURSDAY	HILLS
	FRIDAY	REST
HILLS	SATURDAY	EASY
LONG RUN	SUNDAY	LONG RUN (INC. RACE PACE)
RACE PACE		

NICOLA'S MOST IMPORTANT SESSIONS: LONG RUNS- SCHEDULE THESE FIRST AND SANDWICH BETWEEN EASIER SESSIONS.

NEXT MOST IMPORTANT? THRESHOLD TRAINING — SCHEDULE THIS NEXT, AGAIN, SANDWICHED BETWEEN EASIER DAYS.

HER SCHEDULE ALLOWS FOR AN ADDITIONAL HIGHER-INTENSITY SESSION, WITHOUT COMPROMISING ON RECOVERY, WHICH IS SCHEDULED THURSDAY/FRIDAY.

The reasons for building a programme in this way are, firstly, because it ensures that the most important sessions (the ones you prioritise) don't get missed and, secondly, it forces you to schedule in recovery (in the form of no running, or easy running), rather than leaving it to chance. It also gives your programme a 'hard–easy' pattern, which will lower your chances of injury and ensure you don't end every week feeling exhausted or burned out. And remember the FIT factors (see p. 58) when you are building your programme – don't try to increase too many variables at once or cram in too many high-intensity sessions.

On the opposite page is an example of a training week for Nicola, who is gearing up for a half marathon. This shows you how building a programme works in the real world.

Ring the changes

Once you've got your programme down on paper, bear in mind that you don't have to repeat the same weekly schedule, ad infinitum. Adding variety makes training progressively challenging and stops it from becoming boring and repetitive; it also allows you to address different aspects of fitness at different times.

And remember, even after you've pondered over it, played with it and finally written it down, no training programme is set in stone. If you fail to be flexible about your running and don't listen to your body, you may well end up disillusioned (it was too hard), disappointed (you tried to fit too much in) or injured (it wasn't balanced). Be aware of how your body is responding to your plan and be ready to change it, if necessary.

Weekend warriors

If your lifestyle dictates that you have more time free for running at the weekend than during the week, you can still follow the hard–easy rule (see p. 59) by bending it slightly: do your more demanding sessions on Saturday and Sunday, followed by two easy days on Monday and Tuesday (one of these should be a complete rest day). You could do an additional hard session on Wednesday, with the remainder as easy or rest days.

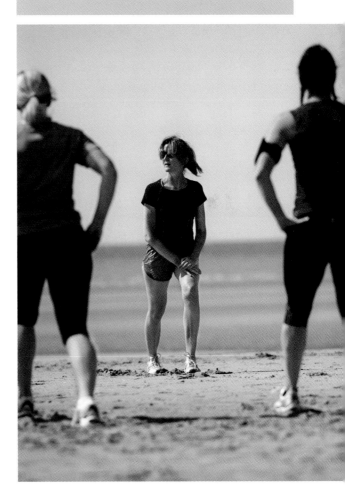

On location
From treadmill to trail

▶▶

I've lived in a big city, a small town, by the sea and deep in the countryside, so I can vouch for the fact that your environment can make a big difference to your running. While most of us would agree that it's more pleasant to run in green surroundings, different running locations and surfaces all have benefits and drawbacks. Being a country dweller can make it difficult to find firm, level surfaces – fine when preparing for a trail race, but not ideal for a swift tempo run. Although there are plenty of quiet roads, many are unlit after dark and pavements are rare. The streets of East London, on the other hand, had pavements and were well lit, but I had issues of personal safety when running at night, whether antisocial behaviour or out-of-

Safety on the roads

The golden rule with traffic is to be seen, but never assume that you have been. I try to make eye contact with a driver before stepping into the road. While jogging on the spot at crossings is tedious, it's far better than taking a risk. I don't recommend doing speed work or timed sessions on routes that involve crossing roads, or you may be tempted to dart across without looking.

In rural areas, the issue is sharing roads with drivers. Always face the oncoming traffic (unless it's a sharp bend, where it may be safer to cross) and wear bright colours day and night (reflectivity is more effective at night – see p. 122).

control dogs. But I had an athletics track nearby. Wherever you live, there will be somewhere to run – most likely a range of options – the key thing is to get as much variety as possible to stop training becoming monotonous and to vary the challenge for your body.

Roads and pavements

The main advantage of road running is that it is readily accessible – most of us have a road (or pavement) going past our door and the surface (although perhaps not the gradient) is probably flat and even. Given that we regularly walk or drive around our neighbourhood, local roads are familiar enough to plan a safe route that meets our needs. Road running is also a little easier than running on more uneven or softer surfaces: if you run along a paved path and then step on to the grass, you'll notice that either your pace slows or your effort level increases. This is because different surfaces have different 'damping ratios' (how much of the energy is absorbed by the surface, rather than returned to the foot). A very soft surface, like sand, will absorb more energy than concrete or tarmac, and requires more effort to push off. On the downside, the journal *Medicine and Science in Sports and Exercise* reports that firmer surfaces are associated with more injuries.

Going off-road

Hear the phrase 'off-road running' and you're likely to picture blazing a trail through scenic wilderness. But running around a football pitch, across a field or on the grass in your local park all qualify as off-road running.

What's the benefit? When you're running off-road,

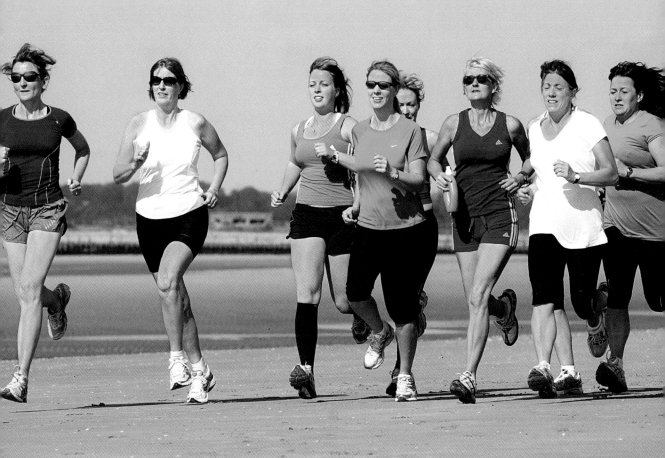

Safety on the trails

- If you're running off-road, always follow the Countryside Code, shutting gates and respecting right-of-way signs.
- Stick to field borders, rather than going straight across, unless signs direct you otherwise.
- Steer clear of livestock (especially cattle, if you are running with a dog).
- Uneven surfaces can put you at greater risk of injuries resulting from slipping or losing footing, so run with a friend or carry a mobile phone.
- Be prepared for changes in weather.

no two 'landings' are identical – you might sink into soft mud or spring off mossy grass, you might need to sidestep a puddle – helping you avoid putting the same forces through the same areas with every step.

Running off-road can also help build strength and stability, by forcing muscles (particularly in the lower leg and ankle) to work harder to keep you upright and stable. This heightens your 'kinaesthetic awareness' – your sense of where your body is in space – making you more nimble on your feet.

Off-road options differ greatly, in terms of their challenge to your fitness and their 'technical' difficulty. A boulder-strewn hill is a far cry from a dusty towpath, requiring greater agility, strength and confidence. While some coaches believe running off-road can help improve your technique, I find it sometimes does the opposite. A really rough trail can cause you to tense up or to run more awkwardly.

If you are new to running off-road, I recommend sticking to more conservative, gentle surfaces to begin with, gradually progressing to more challenging terrain when you feel ready and if it's appropriate to your goals. If you can

maintain the same speed on trail as you can on road, you'll torch considerably more calories (one study found that running through a forest used 26 per cent more calories than a similar-paced road run), but, in reality, most of us adapt our pace according to variations in terrain.

Despite being slightly more demanding than road running, trail running isn't just for fitter runners. Undulating terrain, boggy patches and gates to close all give the perfect opportunity for a breather.

Routefinder

It's easier than you think to leave the roads behind. Here are some suggestions for finding off-road routes:

- Get an Ordnance Survey map to search out potential routes – all public footpaths and bridleways will be marked on this.
- Consider country parks with 'nature walks' or other marked trails. Urban parks can also have areas with natural surfaces like woodchip or dirt trail.
- Canal towpaths are a good bet – and often busy with cyclists and dog-walkers, so you're unlikely to be on your own.

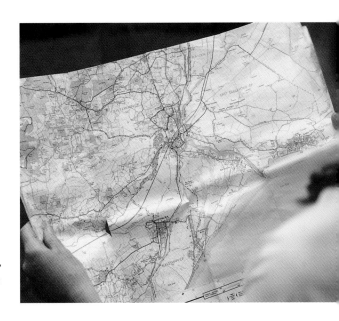

- Are there any long-distance walking routes that pass through your area? London has the Capital Ring and the Green Chain Walk. Check out the National Trails website or look out for footpath signs locally.
- Explore possible routes when walking or cycling, to see whether they'd make a nice run.
- Look up mountain bike trails in your area.
- Rather than doing an 'out and back' route, why not run from home to a local pub or café and get someone to pick you up; or take a train or bus somewhere and run back.

The beach

An expanse of golden sand sandwiched between sparkling sea and sweeping dunes is enough to inspire anyone to break into a canter, but beach running is tough. The energy demand of running on sand is significantly greater than running on grass. It also alters how you run. Research from the University of Western Australia found that running on sand increased cadence (strides per minute), shortened stride length and resulted in a longer ground contact time than a firmer surface. The extent of hip and knee flexion on foot contact was greater and hamstring activation was higher. Overall the beach offers a more challenging workout. But it does have its downsides. Running on cambered (sloped) beaches throws the body out of alignment, while soft sand places extra stress on the Achilles tendon and calf muscles compared to firm, even surfaces, according to the journal *Medicine and Science in Sports and Exercise*. To play it safe, keep your shoes on (a few strides or drills barefoot are fine) and stick to where the sand is wet and more hard-packed. Run both ways: the slope towards the water means that if you only run in one direction, you'll be stressing one side of the body more than the other.

Off-road for beginners

- **Start on grass** More forgiving than concrete and more level and firm than trail, grass can be the perfect surface for your first off-road ventures. Research from the University of Sao Paulo found that natural grass resulted in lower forces through the ball and heel of the foot, compared to asphalt.
- **Changing paces** Running on mixed terrain requires an ability to break your rhythm. On road, you can just get into gear and stay there, but obstacles and uneven terrain dictate your pace and rate of progress.
- **Rate your effort** Trail running is all about effort level, rather than pace, so leave the GPS watch at home and either use heart-rate monitoring, or simply go on your own effort level (see p.66).
- **Look ahead** Try not to keep your eyes glued on your feet, but look at the trail a few metres ahead.

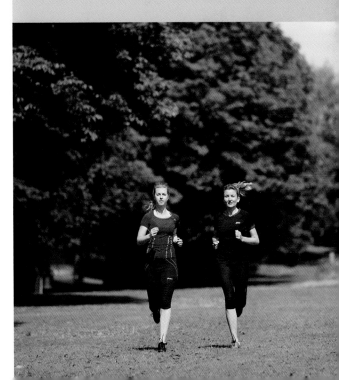

The treadmill

Many women runners take their first steps on the treadmill – and some never venture off it. Although I'd urge every woman to try running outdoors, there are some great advantages to treadmill running, in practical terms and as a training tool. One is being able to avoid running in the cold, wet or dark! Another is feedback. At any given moment, you can check your speed, heart rate, calories per hour, power output, etc. But many of us don't utilise this information. Rather than just counting calories, try monitoring your heart rate at, say, 12kph. After a few weeks of training, see if you can run at the same speed with a lower heart rate.

The treadmill is great for speed work, threshold training and race pace sessions because you can set it to a specific speed. I've used it for a weekly 20–30 minute tempo run for years because it ensures that I maintain my pace – outside it's much easier to let your pace drop off without noticing.

The incline button is another distinct advantage. It offers the perfect place to do hill repeats (running up a given incline a set number of times), or to tackle a hilly run of varying inclines. A study in the journal *Science* found that increasing the incline from 6 to 12 per cent doubled power output.

The treadmill is also fantastic for monthly time trials because the environment is so constant. Warm up first, then select your time or distance and go. Keep a record of your results to monitor progress.

It is also useful if you are returning to running after an injury, as it reduces the impact on your joints and the flat surface minimises the risk of awkward landings or falls. But don't use it all the time, as it isn't exactly the same as free-surface running.

Getting the most out of the treadmill

- Make use of its different functions – don't just get on and start running.

Treadmills vs the great outdoors

Running on a treadmill is not quite the same as running outside. In terms of cardiovascular effort, there's no wind resistance to overcome indoors, and the smooth, flat surface of the belt poses less of a challenge than the more erratic surfaces outdoors. Although the action of running on a treadmill is arguably the same, the mechanics are slightly different, as it's the belt, not your muscles, that's moving your legs, which tends to shorten stride and alter muscle recruitment patterns. Research from Rush University also found that the 'stance phase' of running (when your foot is on the ground) is longer on the treadmill, which isn't desirable.

Even the mental benefits are slightly different – an Australian study found that running outside versus running on a treadmill resulted in less anxiety, fatigue and depression, as well as a higher level of endorphins. So don't rely too heavily on the treadmill for your running fix!

- Limit yourself to one to two sessions per week.
- Make your treadmill runs the shorter or faster sessions.
- Check yourself out! You may be in the rare position of having mirrors in front or to the side of you – use them to check your running technique.
- Don't look down, whether at your feet or at the controls, as this throws the body out of alignment. Glance down occasionally, but try to ensure that you are running tall.
- Set the belt on an incline. Researchers from the University of Brighton recommend setting the gradient to 2 per cent to simulate the great outdoors.

Buying a treadmill

If you don't live near a gym, or prefer to exercise at home, you may want to invest in a treadmill. Think long and hard about how much you will use it before you splash out – it's an expensive piece of equipment, especially if it ends up becoming a glorified rail to hang your clothes on. Consider the following:

- How much space will it need – can you spare the room?
- Think about the view, ventilation and facilities in the room you are planning to use. (You don't want to stare at a wall, or feel as if you are running in the tropics.)
- Never buy before you try. A good store or manufacturer will allow you to test a model before buying.
- Think about functional features. Has it got an incline option? What's the maximum speed? Does it offer pre-set programmes?
- What about style features? Are you happy with a basic control panel or do you want something more complicated? Is a drinks holder important?

Once you have considered these questions, spend as much as you can afford. Choose a decent brand, a model that is sufficiently long and wide, with a nice smooth motion, buttons that are easy to press and a quiet hum.

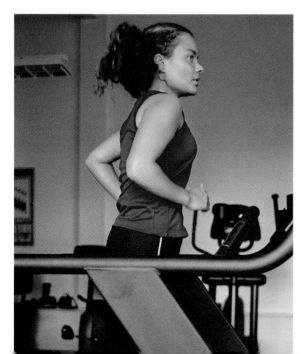

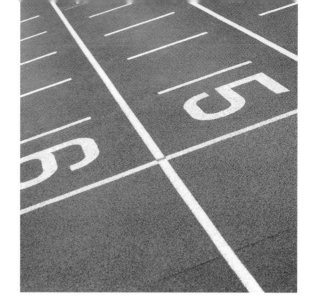

Athletics track

I didn't set foot on an athletics track until I was well into my 20s, but once I did, I fell in love with it. Those straight, white lines, the springy surface and the buzz of activity…

Many people find athletics tracks intimidating, but there's no need to. While there are sprinters tearing up and down, club runners churning out 800m reps and coaches yelling, there are also walkers and runners of all abilities and ambition. Rather than thinking you are entering the world of the serious athlete, see the track as a flat training ground with a good, supportive surface and quantifiable distances.

A track is usually 400m, so four laps equals 1 mile – the perfect distance to test your speed! The other advantage of the track is that you can leave a drink nearby, strip off a layer of clothing and discard it by the side or pop to the loo if you need to. It also allays concerns about personal safety. See Resources, p. 205 to find one nearby.

Track etiquette

- Use the outside lanes if you are walking or jogging. The inside lanes are for runners doing speed work.
- If anyone shouts 'track', move out of their lane as quickly as possible, so they can pass unhindered.
- Always travel in an anticlockwise direction.
- Don't stand around, stretch or leave anything lying on the track.

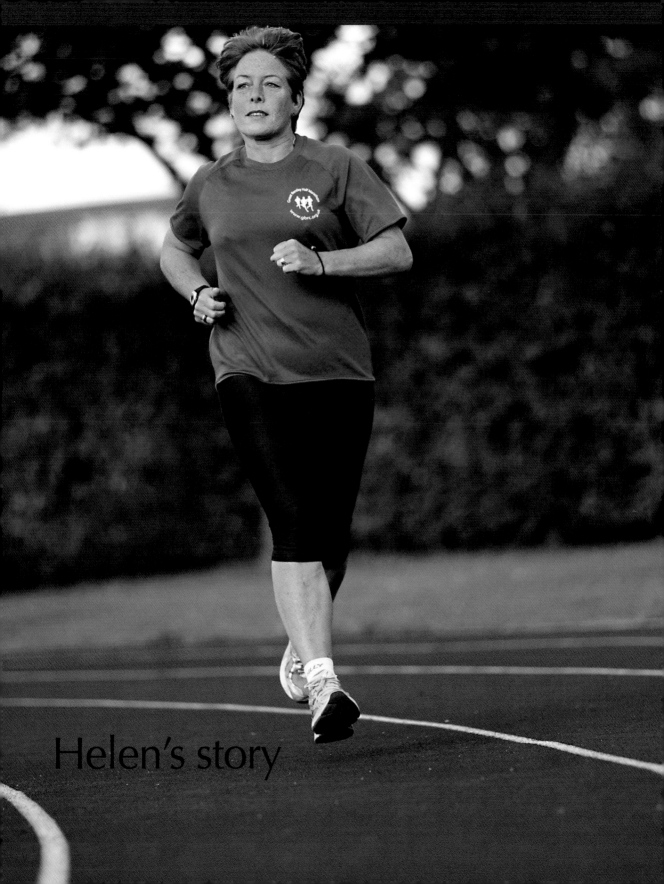

Helen's story

'Enjoy every mile – fast or slow'

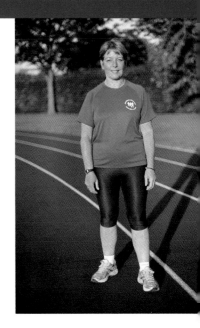

When I started running 12 years ago, at 37 years old, I struggled to run 200 metres. Nowadays, ten miles is my preferred distance. I don't run those ten miles fast, but I run them all the way, from start to finish. Running gives me time to myself – time to think – and inspiration, answers, solutions and acceptance all bubble up while the miles tick over. Being a runner has also given me many great friendships along the way.

Today I ran the 'Tadworth 10' for the fifth time. I consider it the running equivalent of a 'stiff drink': ten tough miles in January, following hot on the heels of the season of feasting and merriment. It had been a tough running year, so I went to Tadworth thinking I would be grateful if I completed the course without a walk. I resolved to take each mile as it came. I knew I was running the race slower than I had in previous years, but somehow, this time, it didn't matter. I have an old Nike T-shirt that claims that 'the essence of running is when both feet are off the ground', and I certainly felt as if I was flying as I careened down the hill at mile eight, revelling in the sheer joy of running for running's sake, the exuberance of putting one foot in front of the other, without time pressures or goals.

Too often, recently, running has felt like self-flagellation, as I dragged myself out the door on yet another long run in too-cold weather, aiming for a specific time over that route, come what may. Far from being an escape, it was starting to feel like one more task on the never-ending to-do list, alongside the ironing, the car insurance, the parking ticket, cooking dinner for four people all going different ways, school work and missing socks.

So I've set myself a new motto: 'Keep it simple.' I don't want to beat myself up when I can't always fit in the training I would need to keep improving my PBs or take all the joy out of running. There are so many things in life to enjoy and running is just one of them – a big, sweaty, healthy one that makes me glow. So I've resolved to enjoy every mile – fast or slow.

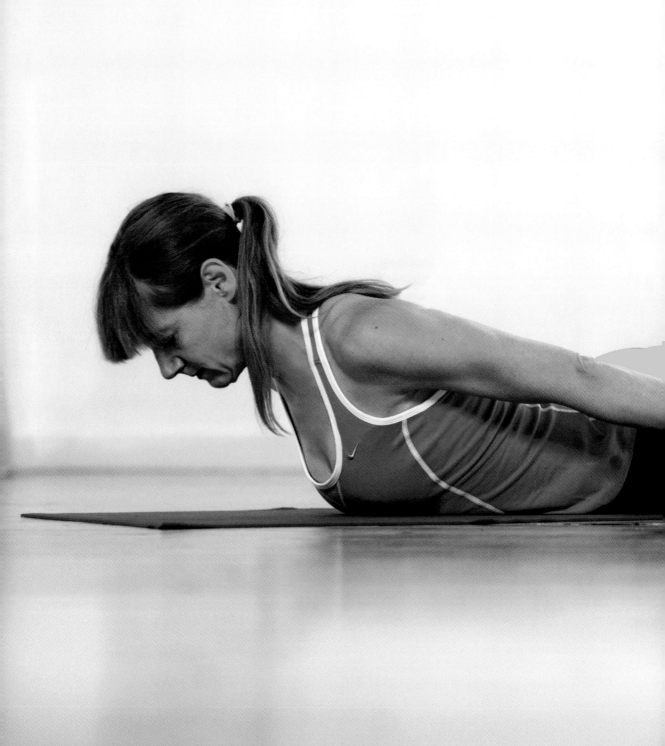

Balancing act

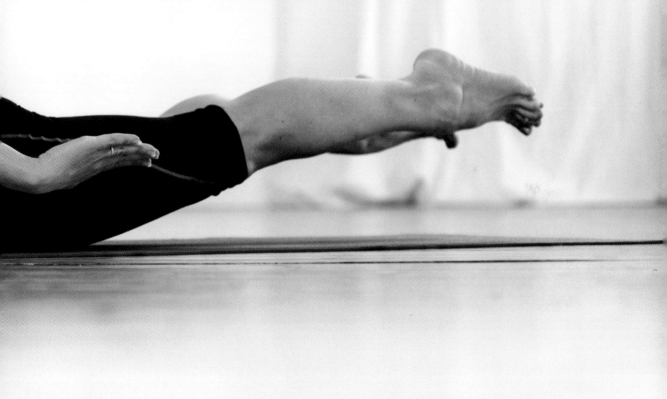

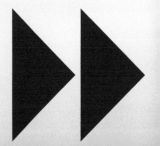

Cross-training

How other activities can improve your running

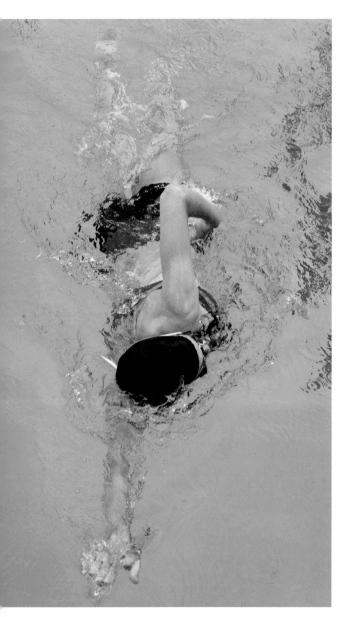

For some women, running is just one component of a varied regime, for others it's their only activity. I used to fall into the second category, but I now believe that whether you are a beginner or a seasoned runner, restricting your physical activity to running is a mistake.

If you need convincing, I'll give you an example. In 2010, I suffered my first running injury in a decade and was sidelined for months. When I looked back through my diary at the preceding weeks, I noticed all other activities – cycling, swimming, strength training – had fallen off the agenda. It's understandable – I was in serious training for what I hoped would be my fastest marathon. But in my keenness to increase my mileage and include plenty of quality sessions, I'd neglected non-running activities. I am convinced this was a contributing factor to my injury.

Why cross-train?

Performing an activity other than your main form of exercise is described as cross-training, but rather than lumping all non-running activities together, I prefer to categorise them according to their purpose:

a) **Cross-training for performance** – an activity that challenges your cardiovascular system like running, but without the impact forces. This would include cross-training during injury, to maintain fitness.

b) **Cross-training for recovery and/or a mental break from running** – this could be something you do because you enjoy it, rather than to benefit your running.

c) **Cross-training that helps your running indirectly** – by improving flexibility, strength, balance or co-ordination. This is the 'behind-the-scenes' work that allows you to run injury-free and with the greatest efficiency. I call this supportive training, rather than cross-training because, in my view, it is an add-on, not an 'instead of'. Strength and flexibility work are crucial for runners.

While the activities in a) or b) might be the same – swimming or cycling, for example – the way you approach them should be different. If the session is meant to substitute a run, make sure the intensity is high enough to be effective and that you know the 'type' of session you are mimicking. Structure it in the same way as you would a run.

If the activity is serving purpose b), make sure that the intensity is gentle – almost effortless – keeping your pace and heart rate low. If you push yourself too hard you risk further exhausting yourself rather than aiding recovery.

Activities that fit b) could also fit c); if you do belly dancing purely for enjoyment, you might find that it also mobilises your lower spine, easing back pain and improving your posture.

So I'm not pigeonholing activities, I'm stressing the importance of having a clear idea why you're doing them, so you can ensure they are fulfilling their purpose. Let's look at the potential of cross-training in more detail.

Cross-training for performance

Running is a high-impact, repetitive activity that places lots of stress on the body. Cross-training allows you to increase the overall volume of your training without adding more miles. Training can be progressed by raising duration or intensity – mixing up your running with cycling or swimming gives you the option to do either.

The more similar an activity is to running, the greater the 'transfer of training' (the benefit to running). This comes down to neuromuscular pathways – the messages nerves send muscles about what to do. The more you repeat a neuromuscular pathway, the more efficient it becomes. An activity with few similarities to running is therefore less beneficial. For the best crossover, seek activities similar to running in terms of muscle usage

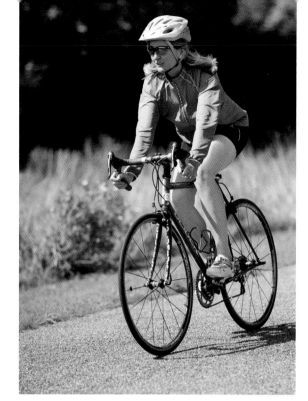

(mainly the lower-body musculature) and movement patterns (forwards, with each leg moving independently).

Research from Trinity College Dublin found that the stair climber and elliptical trainer matched the treadmill very well; over 12 weeks, the fitness gains made by women assigned to one of the three modes of training were the same. Make an elliptical workout more running-specific by using your arms in a running action, rather than holding the handrails.

Cycling also fits the bill, whether indoors (spinning) or outdoors. One study, in the journal *Medicine and Science in Sports and Exercise*, found that when runners added bike interval-training sessions to their usual regime, they improved their 5km times by an average of 30 seconds within six weeks. That's not to say they wouldn't have done so by adding running interval sessions – but that might have tipped the balance of intensity too far. To get your heart rate up to running intensity on a bike, you will probably need to incorporate some hills.

Another running-specific form of cross-training is aqua jogging – running in the pool, using a flotation belt to keep you upright. While the science demonstrates that it's a very effective form of cross-training (it can be as aerobically challenging as running on land because water has greater resistance than air), it's so monotonous that it is generally only used for injured runners. (For more about cross-training during injury, see below).

Swimming uses a greater proportion of total muscle mass than running (because of the upper-body involvement), but since you aren't supporting your own body weight, it isn't such a good calorie burner. And as you are 'weightless' in the water, swimming won't boost bone density in the same way that weight-bearing activity, such as running or aerobics, will. Avoid breaststroke if you've had knee problems, and use proper technique for every stroke. Don't swim with your head above water, which puts extra stress through your neck and spine.

What about walking? The problem is getting up enough speed to make it count. Everyone has a speed at which it becomes easier to run than walk – the so-called 'breakpoint'. Adding hills is an easy way to get your heart rate up, or mix walking and running in your regular training. Walking uses all the major leg muscles, especially the calf and shin, but unless you're climbing steep hills, it doesn't really engage the bottom muscles.

Cross-training during injury and rehabilitation

Sometimes cross-training is our only option – when injury (or a health condition or pregnancy) means we cannot run. In this situation, the activity must not aggravate or stress your existing condition further. This will be dictated by the nature of your problem – some injuries are far easier to work with than others. Back pain can eliminate a number of activities while a calf strain may be fine with most low-impact exercise. Quiz your doctor or physiotherapist about the best activities, but be guided by your body's response: if it hurts, stop.

The goal of cross-training during injury is to maintain, or regain, as much fitness as possible while the problem is resolved. Given that the aim is to return to running, the

Make your cross-training count

- Treat your session like a run with a proper warm-up, cool-down and structure.
- There are theories on how much swimming or cycling 'equals' the same distance in running. (it's estimated that one minute of cycling equals 20 seconds of running), but I recommend training on time and effort level rather than mileage or heart rate. If I do 5 x 3 minutes at RPE level 4 on my bike, with 2-minute recoveries, I feel the same as if I'd done the session running.
- Approach new activities with caution, particularly those with new patterns of movement or muscle groups that don't get used much in running.
- Don't 'discount' your cross-training when planning your programme, or you could end up doing too much.

more specific to running the activity can be the better. That's why aqua jogging is among the most commonly used forms of cross-training among elite athletes. When I took to the pool during my injury, I was wholly unconvinced by aqua jogging – I didn't feel my heart rate was high enough and it didn't feel much like running at all. (Your cadence is significantly slower than on the ground, according to research from the Auckland University of Technology.) But over the weeks, my technique improved and I could work hard enough to get my heart racing. Bear in mind though, that your heart rate will always be lower for the same effort level when exercising in water, so monitor your effort level. To curb the boredom, stick to interval training, rather than steady-paced running. See Resources, p. 205 for suppliers of aqua jogging belts.

The elliptical trainer can be another good option for injured runners. A word of caution: recent research from the National Taiwan University found that although impact was significantly lower (than walking, as well as running), joint flexion angles at knee, hip and ankle were greater, which may not be beneficial in the case of injuries to these particular areas.

Cross-training for recovery

Cross-training can aid recovery from running. Some research shows that gentle activity can be more beneficial than doing nothing in restoring the body's equilibrium. What are good options? It's the intensity that defines an activity as recovery, rather than the exercise itself. Predominantly, you are looking for low- or non-impact activities to allow the joints to recover from the rigours of running. Swimming, Pilates, aqua aerobics, walking and cycling would all be good options. Keep your intensity low and don't overdo the duration – 20–50 minutes is sensible.

Supportive training

I believe that although I could have perhaps staved off my injury by replacing some of my running mileage with cycling or the like, the real problem was the lack of supportive training. As the demands of my running became greater, I needed to be increasing my strength, mobility, flexibility, balance and so on, and instead, I neglected them almost entirely.

Why should it be necessary to do other types of exercise? Weren't we 'born to run'? Well yes, the human body is designed for running, but unfortunately, even those of us who are regularly active spend much of the remainder of our time doing activities our body is less well adapted to, such as sitting for hours, hunching over keyboards or stressing over steering wheels. The result is that we have muscular imbalances – areas that are tighter and weaker than they should be. When we take those imbalances into running, we put ourselves at risk of aches and injuries and compromise our ability to run well.

Take a woman who has been self-conscious about her bust since adolescence. She's developed the habit of folding her arms over her chest, which has dragged the shoulders forwards and let the muscles of the upper back get long and weak. Adopt this posture – with your arms not folded, but shoulders slumped forwards. Now take your arms up into a running action. See what happens? The arms move across the body, rather than back and forth. Do this action with vigour, and you'll feel your torso start to rotate, then your hips will start to move from side to side to counterbalance the torso rotation. Imagine all this happening while you run!

In a woman who sits at a desk all day, the hip flexor muscles will have tightened from being in a shortened position so frequently, while her gluteal muscles will be slack from being continually lengthened. When she begins to run, her pelvis will be tipped forwards by the tight hip flexors, causing an excessive lumbar curve. The weak glutes, unable to stabilise the pelvis on landing, will allow the hips to hitch out to the side and stress the knees and iliotibial bands. In both these scenarios, injury could be just around the corner.

What kind of activities will help redress the balance? Working on flexibility – through mobility exercises and stretching – and improving strength and 'core stability' would come top of my list. The workouts on pp. 100–109 are designed to build running-specific strength and stability and offer a great start, but activities like yoga and Pilates also tick the right boxes.

Whatever supportive training you choose, make sure that you choose something!

Yoga for runners

Yoga is a great way of rounding out a running regime, challenging strength and flexibility, balance and co-ordination. Although running is a symmetrical activity (unlike golf or tennis), it involves only the lower-body muscles and is restricted to a single plane of motion: forwards. Yoga flexes and extends the entire body in every direction so you get a more balanced workout, plus the opportunity to identify potential problem areas, such as tight hamstrings or weak ankle stabilisers. Runners are often drawn to demanding forms of yoga, like Ashtanga or Bikram, but bear in mind that this is meant to be a complementary activity, not another opportunity to exert yourself. I really enjoy my yoga because I don't feel a need to push myself or compete with anyone; I'm there to explore what movements my body can do, other than putting one foot in front of the other.

The focus on the breath in yoga can also be very helpful for runners. In one study, published in *Alternative Therapies in Health and Medicine*, yogic breathing increased lung capacity, while other recent research has found that regular yogis' lung function rivalled that of regular runners.

The following sequence of yoga postures (asanas) has been devised by Laura Denham-Jones, a specialist in yoga for runners. It will supplement and complement your running, helping to prevent and address injuries, by creating strength where you need it and releasing tension where you don't. Yoga is all about finding balance and ease – concentration without tension, effort without struggle. Stay aware of feedback from your muscles and joints while doing the postures and go with, not against, your body. It is normal for your dominant side to be stronger and, therefore, tighter, so feel free to hold postures on that side a little longer. Breathe through your nose to avoid over-straining, keep your eyes soft and focused on one point in space (drishti).

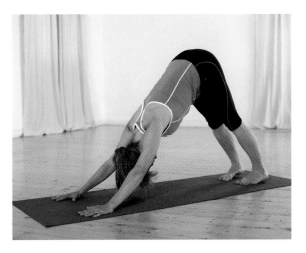

Downward-facing dog (*Adho Mukha Svanasana*)

Why? This pose stretches your hamstrings and calves, strengthens shins, helps to prevent Achilles tendinitis and shin splints, decompresses the lower back and develops upper-body strength.

How? Begin on your hands and knees, hands under your shoulders, knees hip-distance apart. Tuck your toes under and lift your hips up and back, releasing your heels towards the floor and letting your head hang between your hands, bringing your body into an inverted 'V'. Keep your navel gently drawn in and breathe into the back and sides of the ribcage. Bend your knees, if necessary, to avoid rounding the spine. Try bending one knee at a time to stretch the calves. Breathe in this pose for up to one minute.

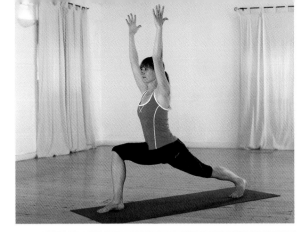

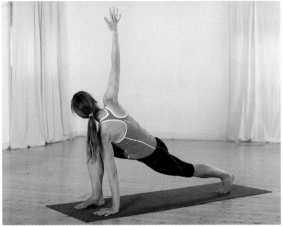

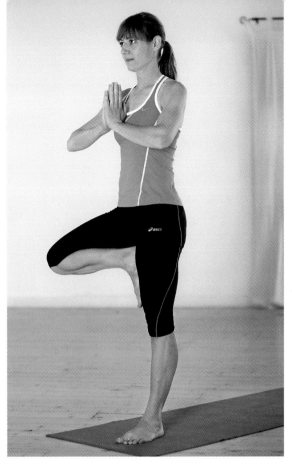

Warrior lunge with a twist (*Virabhadrasana*)

Why? This pose develops stride length and leg strength, by stretching the quadriceps and hip flexors of the back leg and strengthening the glutes and quads of the front leg. The twist increases the stretch in the outer hip of the front leg and strengthens the oblique abdominals.

How? From Downward-facing Dog, step your right foot forwards between your hands, coming into a low lunge. Try to keep the left leg straight by pressing out through the heel. Slowly, bring your body upright and rest your hands on your right thigh, or reach them overhead and look up to challenge your balance. To twist, release your left hand to the inside of your right foot and turn your torso to the right, reaching the right hand up. Keep your hips square and level. To modify this pose, release the left knee to the floor. Breathe in this pose for 30 seconds. Return to Downward-facing Dog and repeat with the left leg.

Tree (*Vrksasana*)

Why? This pose improves balance and focus, strengthens the foot, ankle and knee of the standing leg and teaches the thigh of the lifted leg to rotate in its socket.

How? From standing, shift your weight over your left foot. Pick up the right foot, take hold of your ankle, turn out your thigh and place the sole of your foot on the inner thigh of the left leg. Draw up the thigh muscles of your left leg and squeeze your inner thigh and foot against each other. Look at a point ahead of you and relax your face. Press into the floor with the standing foot and draw up through your belly, reaching up through the top of the head, as though suspended by a string. For a challenge, reach your arms overhead and try looking upwards or closing your eyes. To modify, just bring your right foot to your left ankle. Breathe in this pose for 30–60 seconds. Release slowly and repeat on the other leg.

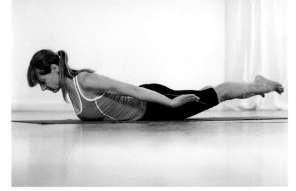

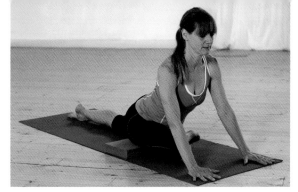

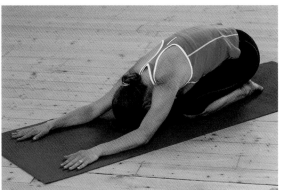

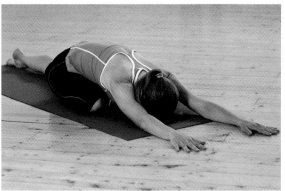

Locust (*Shalabhasana*)

Why? This pose strengthens the upper back, hamstrings and glutes and opens the chest. It teaches the body to extend the leg behind you using your hamstrings and glutes, rather than the lower back.

How? Lie on your front with your hands by your side, palms face up. Draw your navel towards your spine, lengthen your body as if being pulled forwards from the top of the head and backwards through the feet. Keep lengthening and gently lift your chest, legs and arms away from the floor. Avoid raising the chin or over-extending your neck. Stay long and low. Keep your navel drawn in and, if you feel compression in the lower back, tuck your tailbone towards the floor or come down a little. To modify, try lifting the chest only, then the legs only. Breathe in this pose for about 15 seconds. To release, place your palms on the floor under your shoulders, push back to your hands and knees. Then assume 'Child's Pose' by sitting on your heels and reaching your arms forwards with your head on the ground or a cushion.

Pigeon (*Eka Pada Kapotasana*)

Why? This pose stretches the glutes, piriformis (a deep hip rotator) and iliotibial band (ITB) to prevent runner's knee and sciatica, while providing an inner-thigh stretch for the front leg and a hip-flexor stretch for the back leg.

How? From Downward-facing dog (see p. 88) or kneeling, slide your right knee behind your right wrist, place your shin on the floor and take your right foot towards your left wrist. Slowly, begin to walk the left leg back, lowering your hips to the floor. If your hips are tight or your right knee uncomfortable, you may need to place a yoga block or cushion under the right hip. Walk the arms forwards and let your head rest on the floor or a cushion. This can be an intense pose for runners, as there are several deep weight-bearing muscles in the hips that tighten with every foot landing, particularly with an unbalanced gait. Deepen your breath and be patient. Breathe in this pose for one to two minutes. To release, walk your hands back in, roll up and repeat on the other leg.

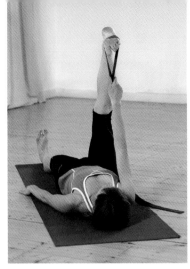

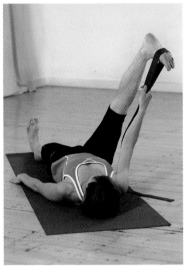

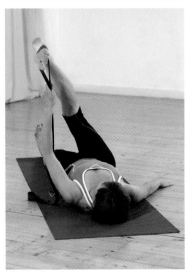

Reclining big-toe hold (*Supta Padangusthasana*)

Why? This pose stretches your hamstrings, groin, outer hip and ITB, for a long, free stride and healthy range of motion.

How? Lie on your back, and take a yoga belt or towel around the sole of your right foot. Extend your left leg out along the floor, reaching out through the heel. If the left leg is buckling off the floor, bend the knee and have the foot on the floor. Press your right heel up towards the ceiling, beginning to straighten your right leg. Press your tailbone down and away as you gently draw your right leg towards you. If the leg begins to shake, ease back.

To develop this pose, turn your right leg out slightly and draw the leg back in the direction of your right shoulder. Return to the centre, then take the belt with the left hand and let the right leg cross the body slightly. Keep the pelvis grounded and evenly weighted throughout. Breathe in this pose for one to two minutes. Release and switch legs.

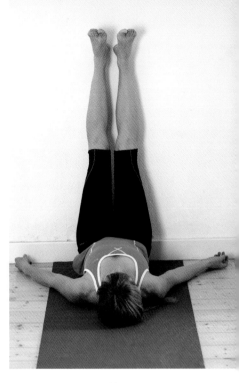

Legs up the wall (*Viparita Karani*)

Why? This pose gently stretches the hamstrings and calves and releases tension in the upper back. Collected lymph fluid in the lower legs drains and circulates, boosting the immune system. Elevation helps to relieve swollen lower legs and assists blood circulation to the upper body after a long time on the feet.

How? Sit sideways with your right hip flush to the wall. Swing your legs up the wall and lower your head and torso to the floor. Shift your hips towards the wall or, if your hamstrings are tighter, you'll need to shift back. Bring your arms to any comfortable position by your sides. Relax legs, shoulders and belly and focus on breathing freely. Maintain this posture for five to ten minutes.

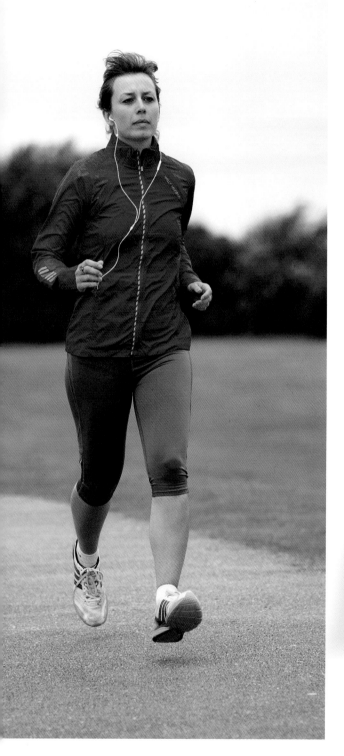

Pilates for posture

Pilates can be another good balancing activity for runners – with a strong emphasis on muscle balance, core stability and posture. Its focus on isolating muscle groups and precise movements make it particularly good for rehabilitation from injury.

The system, which was developed in the early 1900s by Joseph Pilates, can be done in two ways. Studio classes utilise special machines (originally designed by Pilates himself), such as the 'Reformer' and 'Trapeze table', which are equipped with straps, springs and pulleys to facilitate muscle lengthening and strengthening and are often done one-to-one or in very small groups. Or there are 'mat work' classes, which are equipment-free (they often make use of small props, like resistance bands and balls) and take place in a more traditional class format.

> After years of running, I gave triathlon a go. Not only did it give me a new interest and fresh motivation, it also ensured my training was more varied, which had a knock-on effect on my fitness and kept me injury-free.
>
> sam

Stretch yourself
Flexibility for runners

⏵⏵

Running well does not require you to be able to wrap your feet around your neck, but it helps to have a good range of motion in the relevant joints and length and suppleness in your muscles. Limited movement in the ankles, knees or hips can shorten your stride length (it's one of the biggest factors causing runners to slow as they age). Inadequate flexibility may also place unwelcome stresses on other body parts, raising injury risk.

The aims of flexibility training are twofold: to gain or maintain mobility, by regularly taking joints through their full range of motion (dynamic flexibility); and to stretch muscles (passive flexibility) to restore them to their resting length or, if necessary, to encourage them to lengthen.

Dynamic flexibility work is best done before a run because it helps prepare the body for exercise, nourishing cartilage, reducing stiffness and promoting good musculoskeletal alignment. That's why it is an important component of your warm-up. Stretching, on the other hand, is best performed after a run. Running causes muscles to contract and shorten and without regular stretching, they can adapt to this shorter length, compromising efficient movement.

It's important to appreciate the difference between stretching to restore resting muscle length (maintenance) and stretching to gain flexibility (development). After a run, a quick 15–20 second stretch will put you back where you were, flexibility-wise. To improve flexibility you need to hold stretches for longer, or apply specific techniques (see box, p. 94) to enhance their effects. This developmental flexibility training is best done as a stand-alone session after a warm-up, rather than post-run, as you can dedicate more time to each stretch. Yoga is also ideal to work on flexibility – it addresses the whole body and works on strength, balance and co-ordination (see p. 88).

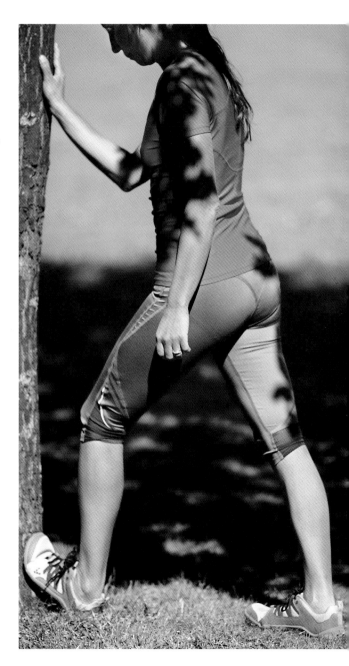

How to stretch properly

1. **Do you know what muscle(s) you are stretching?** You need to know this in order to get the body position right. For example, in a calf stretch, if the back foot isn't pointing directly forwards, the effectiveness of the stretch is compromised.

2. **Do you know how far to take the stretch?** Stretch to the point at which you feel tension and a slight pulling sensation in the muscle, but not pain. Hold this position until the 'stress–relaxation' response occurs and the force on the muscle decreases. Then increase the stretch if you can, and continue to hold. It's helpful to sync your breathing pattern with your stretching: breathe in as you adopt the stretch and exhale as you relax into it.

3. **Are you holding the stretch for long enough?** In a post-run stretch, aim for 15–20 seconds. To develop further flexibility, increase this to at least 30 seconds (some physiotherapists recommend holding stretches for more than a minute, while others advise holding for 30 seconds, but repeating two or three times, which I've found particularly useful on very tight muscles.)

4. **Are you stretching all the muscles you need to?** Many runners overlook important areas when stretching. See pp. 95–97 for a thorough stretch routine.

5. **Bear in mind that flexibility varies from joint to joint.** Just because your hamstrings are nice and loose doesn't mean your hips or glutes are. You may find that you are bendier on one side (if so, stretch the tighter side first, then go back to it after stretching the looser side). Damaged muscle tends to be 'tighter' than healthy tissue, so post-injury, stretches need to be held for longer.

6. **Are you stretching frequently enough?** Some experts believe that you should stretch daily. The benefits of doing so may be great, but it's not something we all have time for, so aim to stretch after every run at least.

Stretch enhancements

- **Facilitated stretching** In a traditional stretch, you assume and hold the position for a prolonged period. This allows the receptors in the muscle to detect changes in length and tension and instruct the muscle to relax to prevent damage. In facilitated stretching techniques, you 'trick' these receptors into allowing a muscle to stretch a little further by resisting the stretch (contracting strongly, but without moving) while simultaneously holding it, or by contracting the opposing muscles.

- **Post-stretch mobility** Stretching aims to encourage a greater range of movement, so it makes sense to apply that newly acquired range immediately. If you've just stretched your quads, then a set of heel flicks (see p. 43) uses those muscles through a bigger range.

- **Foam roller** A foam roller – a large cylindrical slab of firm foam – is a very useful tool for ironing out muscle tightness and tension. It allows you to apply pressure to the muscles and the fascia, realigning muscle fibres, breaking down knots and scar tissue and promoting circulation. Regulate the amount of pressure by using your own body weight. It's particularly useful for tight iliotibial bands (ITB).

The runner's stretch

This stretch routine should be performed after your run, when the muscles are warm. Hold each position for 15–20 seconds. You can also use this as a standalone flexibility workout; make sure you warm up first and hold the stretches for longer, repeating two to three times. The captions describe the stretch for one side, but remember to do them on both sides.

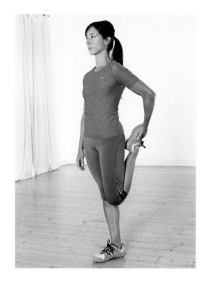

Quadriceps (front of thigh)

Stand tall and take your right foot in your right hand, bringing it towards your bottom. Keep the knees together (don't let the stretching leg splay out to the side) and keep your torso straight, without arching the back. It doesn't matter if your knee is slightly in front of the supporting leg – this just indicates quad tightness. Don't hunch the shoulders!

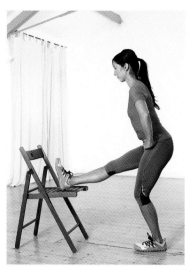

Hamstrings (back of thigh)

Stand in front of a support mid-shin to mid-thigh height (depending on your flexibility) and place your right foot on its surface, with the leg straight. Your support leg should be perpendicular to the ground with the foot facing forwards. Now hinge forwards from the hips until you feel a stretch along the back of the thigh. Don't hunch over.

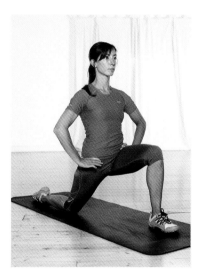

Hip flexors (front of hip)

Take a large step forwards with your left leg, bending the knee and allowing your right knee to rest on the floor, with shoelaces facing down. Bring the torso upright and curl your tailbone under – then gently press the right hip forwards.

Note: it's best to stretch the hip flexors before the hamstrings, to free up the hips.

Hone your hamstring stretch

Since the hamstrings (a group of three muscles) all attach at different points on the pelvic girdle, it's a good idea to vary your position in the hamstring stretch. To emphasise the outer hamstring (the biceps femoris), bring the leg slightly across the midline of your body and rotate the hip joint slightly inwards. To emphasise the hamstrings closest to the middle of the body, turn out at the hip joint and take the leg slightly away from the midline of the body. Finally, slightly bend the leg to shift the focus to the upper portion of the muscles.

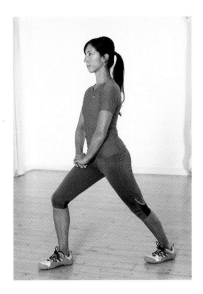

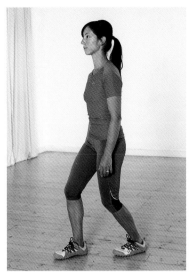

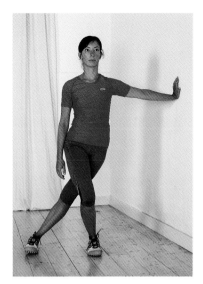

Gastrocnemius (upper calf)

Take a big step forwards with your right foot, bending the knee. Keep the left leg straight, with both sets of toes pointing directly forwards. Gently press the left heel into the ground. Keep the torso upright and don't arch the back. If you don't feel a stretch, take the left foot further back. To accentuate the stretch, visualise 'grabbing' the ground with your toes. Before swapping sides, move on to the soleus and plantar fascia stretches.

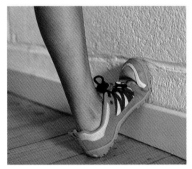

Soleus and plantar fascia (lower calf, Achilles tendon and sole of foot)

Following on directly from the gastrocnemius stretch, take a half step forwards with your left leg and bend both knees, keeping the left heel on the floor. Adjust your weight over the front and back feet until you feel a stretch along the lower part of the left calf. Finally, bring the ball of your left foot up against a wall or stair, bending the knee and gently pressing the foot against the wall. This stretches the plantar fascia under the foot, too.

Abductors and ITB (outer hip)

Stand to the left of a wall or pole and take your left leg behind the right leg, sliding the foot away. Supporting yourself with your left hand, lean well into the hip of the left leg, feeling a stretch through the left hip. (You may feel a stretch along the side of the left thigh, but the ITB doesn't have many nerves in it, so you are more likely to feel the 'pull' in the hip.)

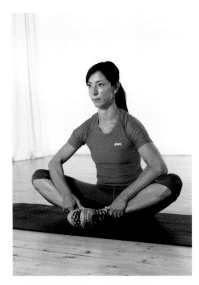

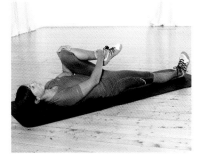

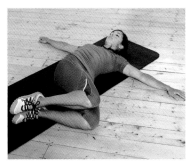

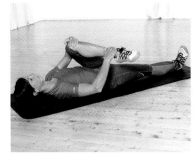

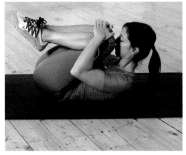

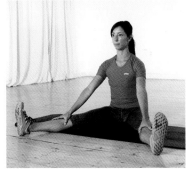

Adductors (inner thighs)

Sit tall (you can sit against a wall if your pelvis wants to tilt backwards), bend the knees and bring the soles of your feet together, or as near as you can without slumping back. Gently press the knees open with your hands and hold. Now extend the legs out straight, opening them as wide as you can without creating tension. If this is comfortable, hinge forwards from the hips to increase the stretch.

Gluteals and piriformis (bottom and hip rotators)

Lie flat on the floor and take hold of your left leg around the knee, drawing it towards your chest. Feel a stretch in the bottom. Now bring your knee slightly towards your right shoulder and, taking hold of the ankle, gently draw the shin to the right – you should feel this in the hip rotator muscles, deep in the left hip.

Erector spinae (lower back)

Lie with your knees bent and feet flat on the floor, close to your bottom. Open your arms at shoulder height and, keeping your shoulders on the floor, let the knees drop down to the left. Draw them back to the centre and drop to the other side. Do this a few times and finish by hugging the knees into the chest.

Be strong
Why strength and stability matter

▶▶

Strength training is part of every elite athlete's training regime, but for many of us – already hard-pressed to find time for running – it barely gets a look-in. It's a pity, because being strong helps keep injuries at bay and yields improvements in efficiency and speed. A recent study review from the University of Connecticut found that strength training improved running economy by an average of 4.6 per cent and boosted race times in elite runners. The benefits for amateurs are likely to be even greater.

What do we mean by strength? There's a difference between a muscle maintaining or repeating a low-level contraction over a long period and exerting its maximum force in one go. The first scenario is more correctly called muscular endurance, while the second is muscular strength – both are important to runners.

Here's an example: the muscle at the top of the hip (the gluteus medius) helps keep the pelvis level and stable while we run. This doesn't take a lot of force, but it does need to maintain pelvic stability over a prolonged period. Meanwhile, the gluteus maximus, the biggest muscle in the bottom, extends or 'drives' the hip backwards.

Some muscles are cut out to be stabilisers while others are there to create movement. You may think working the 'mover' muscles would be more useful to a runner – stronger means more powerful, faster. But if your stabilising muscles can't maintain good posture, then these mover muscles aren't as well placed to do their job. If you can't stabilise your pelvis standing still on one leg, how are you going to do it running for half an hour? The body will cleverly find a way of compensating to enable you to continue running. But over time, these compensations can create muscular imbalances, wear on the joints and even injury. It pays to address stability and strength – in that order.

The core issue

You have probably heard of the term 'core stability'. It is used to refer to the stabilising muscles in the trunk area, which form an 'internal corset' around the abdominals and lower back, protecting the spine and maintaining posture. If these muscles are strong enough, they provide a great launch pad for the legs to work from, but if they are weak (and sedentary living, especially constant sitting, tends to weaken them), this can cause biomechanical problems anywhere from the lower back down. But we don't only have stabilising muscles in the trunk – we have them throughout the body.

The hotspots for runners are the ankle, knee, pelvis and trunk. Weakness in any of these areas can affect that joint's function or have a knock-on effect elsewhere.

The workout over the page is designed to work these muscles, improving your posture and balance and reducing your risk of injury, as well as laying the foundations for more demanding exercises to improve performance and running economy.

Use the tests shown to assess your stability and the recommended exercises from the workout to improve. Alternatively, complete the whole workout for a few weeks before progressing to the running-specific strength workout on p. 106. You could also combine stability exercises for your 'trouble zones' with more dynamic moves to enhance your strength. Aim to do some core training at least twice a week. Even five to ten minutes is worthwhile, before or after a run.

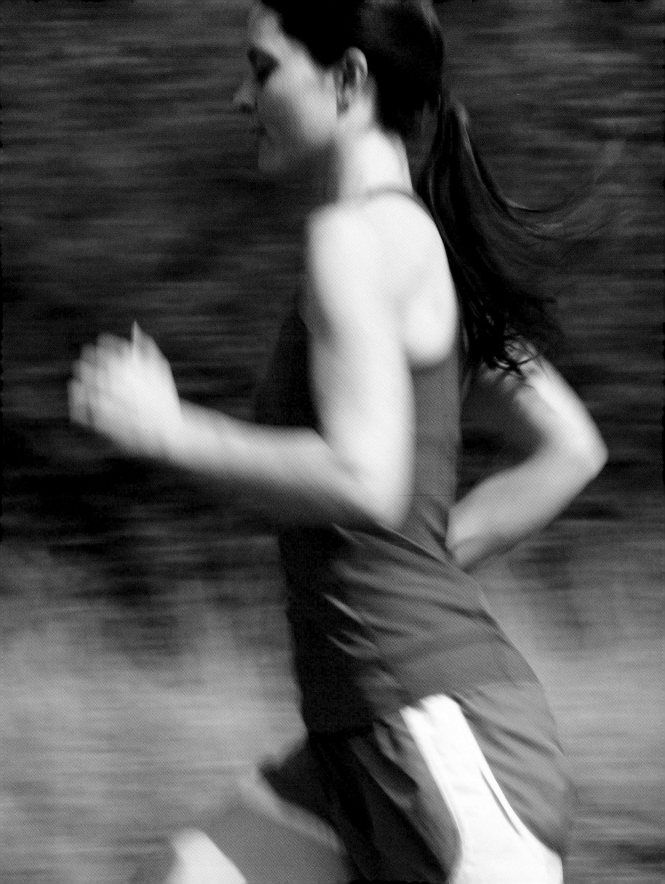

The tests

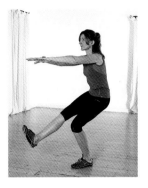

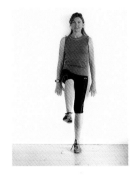

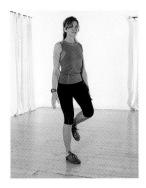

Single-leg dip: to assess knee stability

Stand on one leg with your body tall and centrally aligned. Bend the knee of the support leg to create a 90-degree angle at the back of the knee joint. If your knee rolls inwards, rather than staying directly over your middle toe, this indicates that your knee is maltracking. The kneecap sits inside a little ridge in the knee joint and correct alignment enables it to travel smoothly up and down this ridge. But if the iliotibial band (ITB), which runs along the side of the leg from the hip to just below the knee, is tight, or if there is an imbalance in the muscles along the front of the thighs, the kneecap can be pulled slightly off kilter, causing irritation under the kneecap and on the lateral side of the knee. A staggering 40 per cent of running injuries are knee-related.

Needs work? Try exercises 5, 7 and 9

Wall stand: to assess pelvic stability

Stand with your feet about 7.5cm away from a wall and lean against it. Lift one leg by bending the knee to approximately 90 degrees. If you feel yourself shift to the other side, or if your hip drops on the opposite side, you are almost certainly lacking strength and stability around the hips and pelvis. This is often a weak area in runners, as the muscles that perform these actions get strong through lateral or side-to-side motion, which you don't do much in running. The result is that the ITB takes over and ends up shortening and tightening.

Needs work? Try exercises 1, 4 and 10

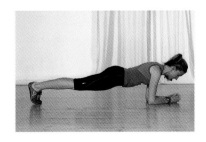

The stork: to assess ankle stability

Stand tall, with feet close together and arms by your sides. Lift one foot, keeping the support leg straight (not locked) and the body erect. Can you hold for 20 seconds without wobbling?

Needs work? Try exercises 6 and 8

The plank: to assess trunk stability

If you've ever been told not to 'sit in your hips' (see p. 48) when you're running, you may need to improve your strength and stability around the core. Lie face down with elbows under shoulders and forearms and palms on the floor. Engage the core and raise your body up to form a straight line from the nape of the neck to the heels. Hold, but don't forget to breathe. Can you hold for 45 seconds?

Needs work? Try exercises 2, 3 and 10

Stability workout for runners

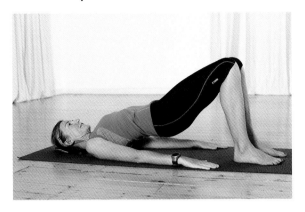

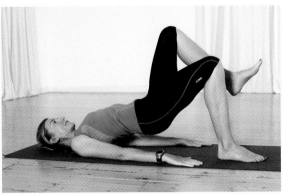

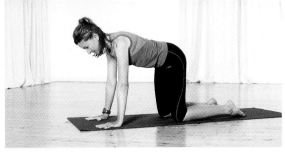

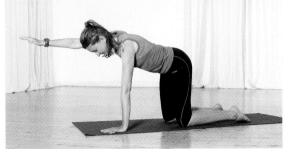

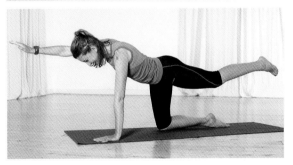

1. Bridge

Aim: to strengthen the glutes and lower back and improve pelvic stability. Helps to prevent 'sitting in the hips'.

Lie on the floor with knees bent and feet flat. Curl the spine off the floor to form a straight line from knees to shoulders. Hold for five seconds, then return the spine to the floor, aiming for the back to curl down bit by bit and the buttocks to hit the floor last. Repeat ten times. Progress to five ten-second holds. Once you do this comfortably, lift each foot alternately off the floor (just a few centimetres) in a slow 'marching' action, aiming for 20 steps. But make sure the pelvis stays level and does not tip from side to side. (You can place your hands on your hipbones to check this.) Repeat three times.

2. Abdominal hollowing

Aim: teaches you to draw in the deep abdominal muscles without restricting your breathing or 'bracing' the entire abdominal region.

Start on all fours with knees under hips and hands under shoulders. Maintain the spine's natural curves and completely relax your abdominal muscles. Now engage the pelvic floor (as if you were trying to stop yourself weeing) and gently draw in the lower part of the tummy (imagine doing up the zip on your jeans) without moving your ribcage, tensing up or allowing your back to move. Hold for ten seconds, breathing freely. Build up to ten repetitions.

To progress: perform the exercise as above, but slowly lift one hand and extend the arm in front. Hold for five seconds and then repeat on the other side. When you can do this, lift the opposite arm and leg simultaneously.

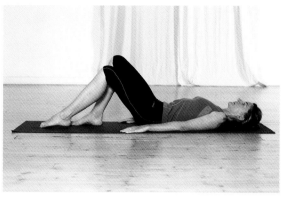

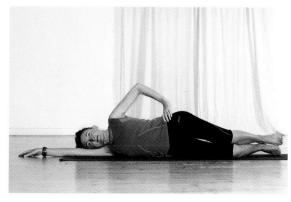

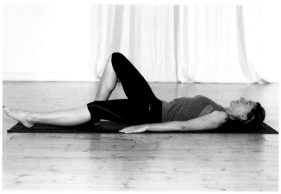

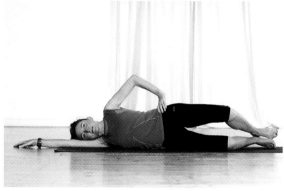

3. Leg slide

Aim: to maintain a stable core while the legs move.

Lie on your back with knees bent and feet flat on the floor. Engage your abdominals (see Abdominal hollowing p. 101) and, maintaining this contraction, slowly slide one foot away from you along the floor until the leg is straight. Pause, then draw the foot back to the start position and repeat with the other leg. Aim for ten repetitions per leg.

4. Clam

Aim: to activate and strengthen the gluteus medius and deep hip rotators, preventing the hips from dropping side to side in running.

Lie on your side, with hips stacked one on top of the other and hips and knees flexed. (Your heels, bottom and back should all be in line.) Make sure the back is not arched. Leaving the feet together, slowly lift the top knee by turning out at the hip, but only go as far as you can without letting the pelvis or back twist. Hold for five seconds, then lower and repeat. The more bent the legs, the easier, so gradually move the heels further away from you. Aim for ten repetitions per side. Progress to five ten-second holds.

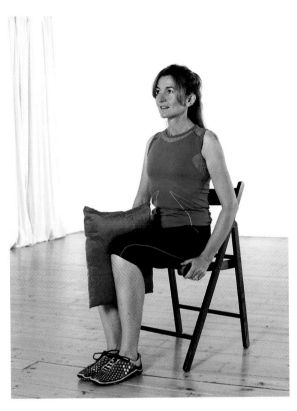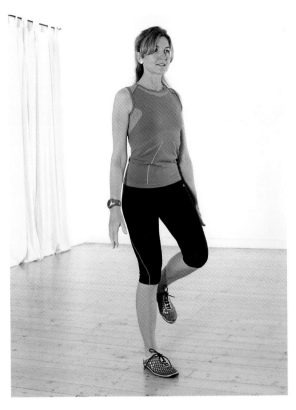

5. Cushion squeeze

Aim: This exercise works the vastus medialis obliquus (VMO; the weakest link in the quad group), the inner thighs (adductors) and the all-important gluteus medius. It can help you avoid or deal with knee problems.

Sit on the edge of a firm chair with feet flat on the floor and place a cushion between your knees. Squeeze your bottom and inner thighs simultaneously, holding the contraction for ten seconds before slowly releasing it. Build up to six repetitions.

6. Stork

Aim: to strengthen the lower leg stabilisers, improve balance and proprioception (awareness and 'feedback' from the ground)..

Stand on one leg with the other leg slightly bent and arms by your sides. Hold for 20–30 seconds. If this is easy, do it with your eyes closed. When that gets easy, try some very low hops on the spot – 20 jumps on each side, aiming to stay in the same position by maintaining good posture. Don't look down!

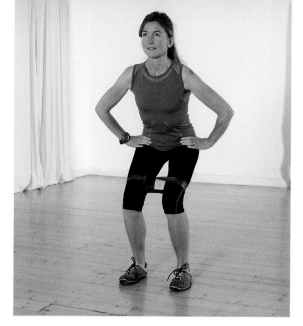
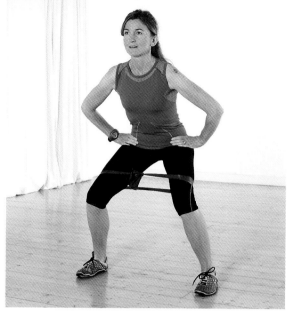

7. Lateral stepping

Aim: to balance hip strength by working the hips through abduction and to improve hip, knee and ankle alignment. This is a good exercise for runners with 'runner's knee' (patellofemoral pain syndrome).

Secure a resistance band around your thighs, just above the knees. Stand with feet below hips and drop your bottom towards the ground, bending the knees into a squat. Maintaining the squat, step directly to the side, ensuring your toes face forwards and not out to the side. Bring the other foot alongside the first one, then step out again with the first foot. Do five steps in one direction and then five back in the other, leading with the other foot. Repeat three times.

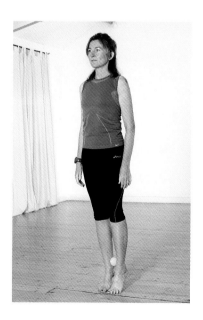
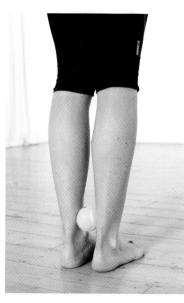

8. Stability raises

Aim: to strengthen the tibialis anterior muscle and ankle stabilisers, reducing the risk of shin, ankle and foot problems.

Place a tennis ball or similar between your ankles, just above the ankle bones and *gently* hold it in place. Ensure your feet are pointing directly forwards. Rise up on to your toes, pause and lower slowly, maintaining your balance. Don't allow the feet to roll out towards the little toes as they rise up – if you do, the ball will fall out. Aim for 12–20 repetitions. Repeat three times.

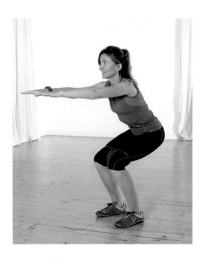

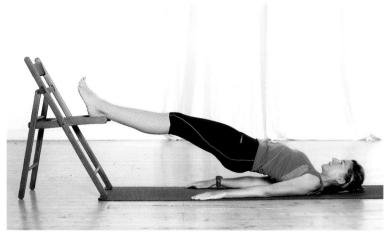

9. Resisted squat

Aim: to improve knee, hip and ankle alignment and strengthen the quads, hamstrings and hips.

Stand with feet hip-distance apart and a resistance band secured above the knees with some tension in the band pulling your knees together. Have your arms extended in front at chest height. Take your bottom backwards and, bending the knees, squat until your thighs are at or near parallel, pushing out against the resistance band to prevent the knees rolling inwards. Do not overarch the back and try to keep the torso upright. Pause in the lowered position then stand up and repeat. Aim for two sets of ten repetitions.

10. Straight-leg pillar

Aim: to strengthen the back, glutes and hamstrings, to improve hip drive and prevent the torso tipping forwards in running.

Lie face up on the floor with your heels resting on the bed or a chair (a higher surface is easier than a lower one). Push your heels down into the surface and raise your hips to form a straight line (don't let the hips sag or the back arch). Hold for five seconds, then slowly lower almost to the floor and repeat. Aim for ten repetitions. Progress to five reps of ten seconds.

Give me strength

Once you have good core stability, you can begin to target your strength training more towards performance, rather than injury prevention. It's thought that strength training enhances neuromuscular pathways, leading to more efficient muscular contractions and the ability to exert or resist greater forces. It also fortifies the ligaments and tendons and boosts bone health. But what kind of strength training gives the best results?

I recommend focusing on running-specific exercises – ones which use the muscles in the same way as running. There is a lot of 'eccentric contraction' in running – contractions in which the muscle is lengthening rather than shortening. You can mimic that in your strength training. In running you bear weight on one leg at a time, so you can replicate that. And you use multiple muscle groups at once – so you don't want to include exercises that isolate a specific muscle group. That's why exercising with your own body weight, or using 'free weights' is better than using machines.

Strength workout for runners

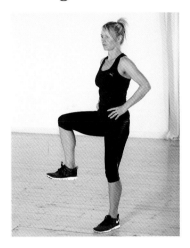 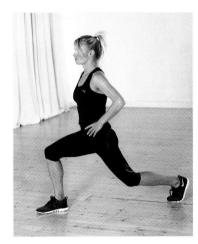

1. Stepover lunge

Aim: to strengthen the hip flexors, quads, hamstrings and glutes and challenge balance. The inner and outer thigh muscles stabilise you.

Stand tall with feet below hips. Lift one leg and raise it to 90 degrees, without letting the torso tip to the other side, the hip 'hitch' out or the support leg bend at the knee. Pause for two seconds, then take a big step forwards into a lunge, allowing the back heel to come off the floor and the back knee to travel towards the floor. Keep the torso upright and the spine in neutral (do not arch the back). Do not extend the front knee beyond the toes. Push back through the front foot to return to standing. Aim for 10–16 repetitions. Repeat on the other side.

Make it count

- Start with one set of each exercise and stick with the lower end of the suggested repetitions. Increase to two sets when you feel ready.
- As exercises get easier, increase the number of repetitions or add weight in the form of dumbbells or resistance bands to increase the challenge.
- Strength train on easy-run or rest days and don't do strength workouts on consecutive days.
- Aim to train twice or three times per week.
- Don't neglect the non-running muscles. I haven't included upper-body exercises here but they will help to balance out your regime.
- Consider getting a running coach or personal trainer to devise a strength workout for you and to ensure that you are using the correct technique.

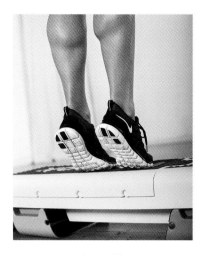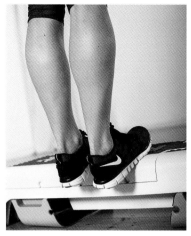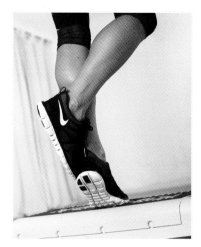

2. Eccentric calf raise

Aim: to improve lower-leg muscle balance and strengthen the calf through the lowering phase, when it works hardest during running. This is used in the prevention and rehabilitation of Achilles and calf problems.

Stand on a stair or step with just the balls of your feet on the surface, the heels extending over the edge. Rise up on to the balls of both feet and then drop down quickly. Work through your full range. To progress, press up with both feet but lower with just one foot at a time. Aim for 10–16 repetitions.

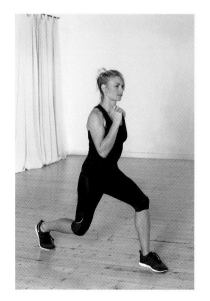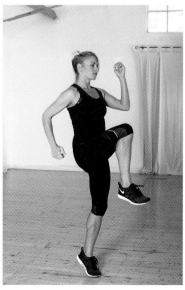

3. Knee drive

Aim: to strengthen each leg independently and provide a stability challenge.

Take a biggish step backwards with your right leg, and bend both knees, allowing the right knee almost to reach the floor, and ensuring the left knee doesn't extend over the toes (you should be able to look down and see your toes). Try to keep the torso upright and the pelvis level. Then drive your right knee up and through to the front before stepping immediately back into a lunge. Aim for 10–16 repetitions. Repeat on the other leg.

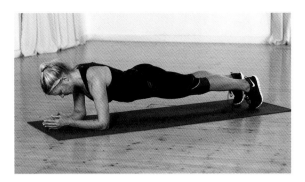

4. Plank

Aim: to promote good running posture by strengthening the core stabilisers and lower back with the body fully extended.

Lie face down on the floor. Engage the core and, supporting yourself on your forearms and feet, raise your body up to form a straight line from the nape of the neck to the heels. Hold, but don't forget to breathe. Progress by extending the length of the hold, building up towards one minute. Or combine the plank and side plank (below) into one exercise (front, side, front, other side, front – 15 seconds per position).

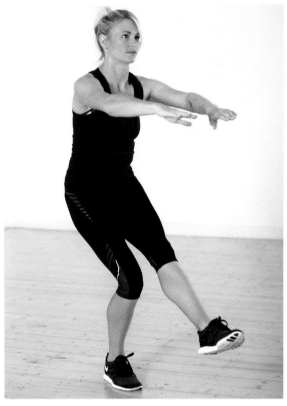

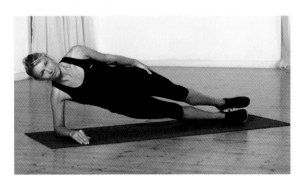

5. Side plank

Aim: to strengthen the lateral stabilisers in the trunk region.

Lie on your side, supporting yourself on the elbow and forearm, with your legs stacked and body aligned (make sure your bottom isn't sticking out). Keeping navel pulled to spine, raise up on to the elbow. Visualise trying to keep the lower side of your waist lifted away from the floor. Progress by extending the length of the hold – building up towards one minute. Or combine with plank as detailed above.

6. Single-leg dip

Aim: to strengthen the muscles that stabilise the pelvis and support the knee, preventing the knees from rolling in during running.

Stand tall with feet below hip bones and hands extended in front of you. Lift one foot in front of the body and then 'sit down' by flexing the hip and knee of the supporting leg. Lead with the bottom, not the knee. Keep the hip bones level and torso upright, and make sure the bending knee travels in line with the middle toe and does not roll inwards or outwards. Lower as far as you are able to, pause and straighten. Do 8–12 repetitions then change sides.

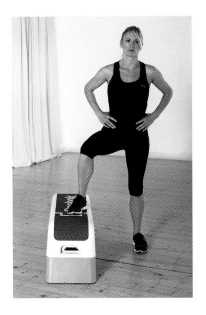
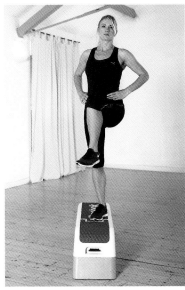

7. Lateral step-ups

Aim: to strengthen the quads, hamstrings, glutes and calves through a non-linear range of motion.

Stand side-on to a bench or step, with your right foot placed upon it, knee bent to approximately 90 degrees. Take your weight on to the right foot and straighten the leg, driving up with your left knee at the same time. Take the left foot back to the floor and repeat immediately. Aim for 10–16 repetitions. Repeat on the other side.

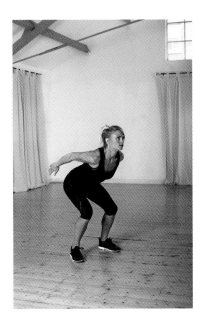
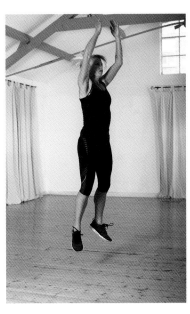

8. Squat jumps

Aim: to strengthen all the running muscles and improve their elasticity and power.

Start in a squat position, with feet hip-width apart and knees aligned over feet. Keep the torso upright. Spring up into the air as high as you can (you can use your arms for momentum). As you land, immediately return to the squat position and go straight into the next jump. Aim for 8–12 repetitions.

Staying healthy
Running free of injuries

▶▶

Eavesdrop on a group of runners and you'd be forgiven for assuming that as far as injuries are concerned, it's not a matter of if, but when. Depending on which studies you read, the prevalence of injuries among runners for any given year ranges from 50 to 75 per cent. Although many of these can be put down to biomechanical or technique faults – like knees that roll in or overstriding – many sports injury experts believe the majority of injuries are caused by 'training errors', such as running on hard surfaces too often or increasing mileage too quickly. That's good news, because it means such errors can be avoided, and injury risk lowered. As discussed in Chapter 3, even biomechanical efficiency can be improved, reducing the likelihood of problems occurring in the first place and, just as importantly, recurring.

Injury is not inevitable and many of the common problems that plague runners are preventable. My ten rules for staying injury-free are below; most direct you to other sections for further information because in a sense, every aspect of smart training is geared towards two things: reducing injury risk and enhancing performance.

The ten rules of injury prevention

1. Don't overdo it. Trying to achieve too much, too quickly is the most common error among runners – especially new ones – both in terms of the overall volume of running and the rate at which they progress. I discuss the principle of progressive overload on p. 58 – the notion that to progress successfully, you need to gradually increase your workload. Every runner has their own threshold, beyond which their likelihood of getting injured increases, no matter how gradually they increase their mileage. Unfortunately, we tend only to discover our threshold by crossing it. Just because your friend does 60 miles a week and stays injury-free, it doesn't mean that you can or should do the same.

2. Schedule rest days. It is during rest, not exercise, that your body gets fitter and stronger, adapting to your training. If you don't rest enough, you are never allowing your body to adapt, and you won't reap the full benefits. Research from the University of Nevada found that fatigue reduced runners' ability to deal with impact forces by a factor of 12 per cent, increasing the likelihood of injury. According to research in the journal *Running Research News,* reducing the number of runs done on consecutive days lowers injury risk, even when overall mileage stays the same, because it allows more recovery time between sessions. That's why the hard–easy rule works so well – it forces you to schedule easy days (rest days or easier runs) around tougher ones. If you take part in races, ensure you include sufficient recovery post-event.

Red flags

Seek advice from a sports medicine expert before you embark on a running programme if you have just had a baby, have a pre-existing injury or trouble spot, back pain or an unusual running gait. You may want to have a pre-running 'MOT' in the absence of such problems; many physiotherapists and sports injury clinics now offer this kind of service.

3. **Warm up and start slowly.** There is plenty of evidence that when done correctly, warming up reduces your injury risk. By preventing a sudden accumulation of lactic acid in the muscles, it helps you to ease into a run more comfortably (see p. 42).

4. **Maintain good flexibility.** Although there's no evidence that one stretch session in isolation will reduce your injury risk, in the long term, staying flexible through regular stretching does appear to have an impact. See p. 93 for more information on flexibility and a stretch routine for runners.

5. **Be strong**. Fitness is about balance, and focusing only on endurance is like tuning a car's engine while ignoring the flaking paintwork. Building strength and resilience in your muscles and connective tissues is a great way to offset potential damage. A study in 2007 from the University of Calgary put a group of runners with knee, ankle and foot pain on to a hip-strengthening programme for six weeks. By the end of the study, 90 per cent were pain-free. Having appropriate strength will help you run faster and make your muscles more fatigue resistant; it can help to improve your technique too. See pp. 98–109 for strength and stability workouts.

6. **Vary your surfaces and terrain.** I do a lot of my running off-road in order to reduce overall forces through my joints and allow more variability between footstrikes. There's even a significant difference in the 'give' of asphalt (roads) compared to concrete (paths and pavements), which is much less forgiving. Take care to avoid running on cambered roads, as this can irritate the iliotibial band. Read more about running surfaces on pp. 74–79.

7. **Wear good shoes**. While no pair of shoes can guarantee you'll stay injury-free, wearing worn-out trainers won't help. The lifespan of a running shoe is surprisingly short – approximately 300–500 miles. If you're running 30 miles a week, that's only around 10–16 weeks. I've had many a runner guiltily admit that they've had their running shoes 'a few years'. It's also important that you have shoes that are appropriate for you and your type of running. Read more in Chapter 6.

8. **Strike a balance.** Whether it's too many long runs or running too fast, an unbalanced programme can raise your risk of injury. For the types of sessions to include in your programme see p. 61 and for how to construct a balanced schedule see p. 70.

9. **Never run through pain**. Pain is your body's way of telling you something is wrong. So listen to it! If you ignore it, then what could have been cured by a day or two's rest, a good sports massage or an ice pack, could end up being an injury that sets you back far longer. Rest should be your first port of call, but that doesn't mean doing nothing other than waiting and hoping that the problem will go away… For how to be proactive about niggles and injuries, see Chapter 9.

10. **Work on your technique.** Some coaches have an 'If-it-ain't-broke-don't-fix-it' attitude to running technique, meaning that if your running style hasn't caused you injury so far, don't change it. But what you may be able to get away with when you are running three times a week may not be the same as what you can get away with when you up your mileage or when you are five years older. I always think it's worth addressing shortfalls in your technique – it might not only keep you out of the sports injury clinic, it could also help you run faster and more efficiently. Find out more about running technique on pp. 46–55.

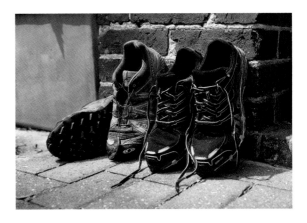

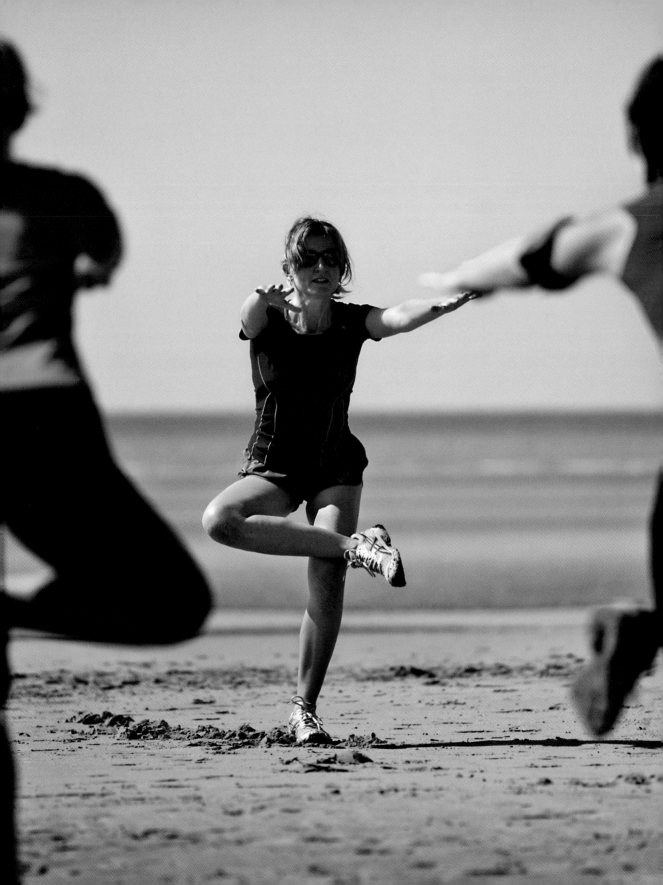

There's the rub

Sports massage is widely used to help recovery and is part of every elite athlete's regime. Regular treatments allow a good therapist to spot any problem areas that, if left untreated, could develop into full-blown injuries, making a great 'early-warning system'. Sports massage is a far cry from a relaxing Swedish massage; it works very deeply into the tissues, easing out knots and tightness and promoting fresh blood supply. It can be uncomfortable or even painful. It used to be believed that sports massage worked by flushing lactic acid out of the muscles, but it is now known that muscle soreness isn't caused by a build-up of lactic acid but by microscopic damage to the muscle fibres. Massage, through breaking down fibrous tissue and adhesions, can help promote healing and hasten recovery.

I've certainly found sports massage invaluable, particularly when I'm in marathon training. Once a month, or more, is ideal. Otherwise, try to schedule the odd treatment for a couple of days after a long or hard run. You can also DIY: work from foot to hip with firm strokes (one hand on top of the other enables you to use more force). If you find a tight spot, massage gently for a few minutes and then apply light to medium pressure, holding for a few seconds before gently stretching out that area. Avoid rubbing bony areas, and stay away from sites of injury – incorrect treatment could make it worse. See Resources, p. 205 to find a sports massage therapist.

Right on Q

You'll often hear it said that women are more at risk of knee and hip injuries because of their larger 'Q angle' (the direction of pull of the thigh muscle on the kneecap). If you are a classic pear-shaped woman, you may well have a wide pelvis and, therefore, a larger-than-average angle between where your thigh bone originates and your knee joint. This tends to be associated with a low knee pick-up when running and the classic girlie 'heel flick' to the side. While you can't do anything about your skeletal structure, ensuring that you maintain strength and flexibility will minimise injury risk. Tight hip flexors and weak glutes are common problem areas, so ensure you stretch and strengthen these muscle groups (see p. 95 and p. 101).

"

I'd been spending so much time 'training', that I'd forgotten to take time for the gentler things, such as stretching. Ten minutes of yoga every day is starting to pay off as I'm creaking far less and have stopped feeling like I'm getting too old for running!

sarah H

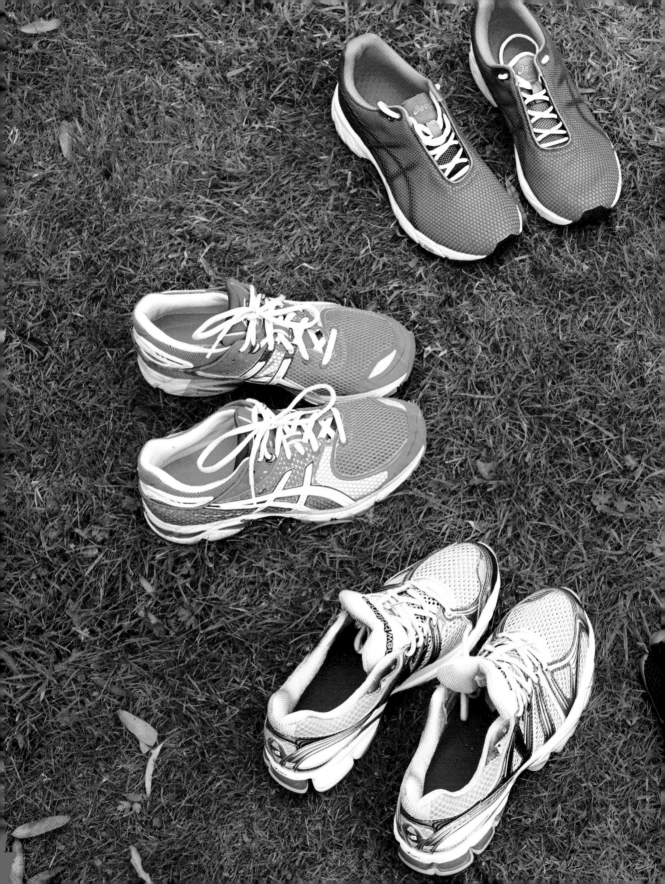

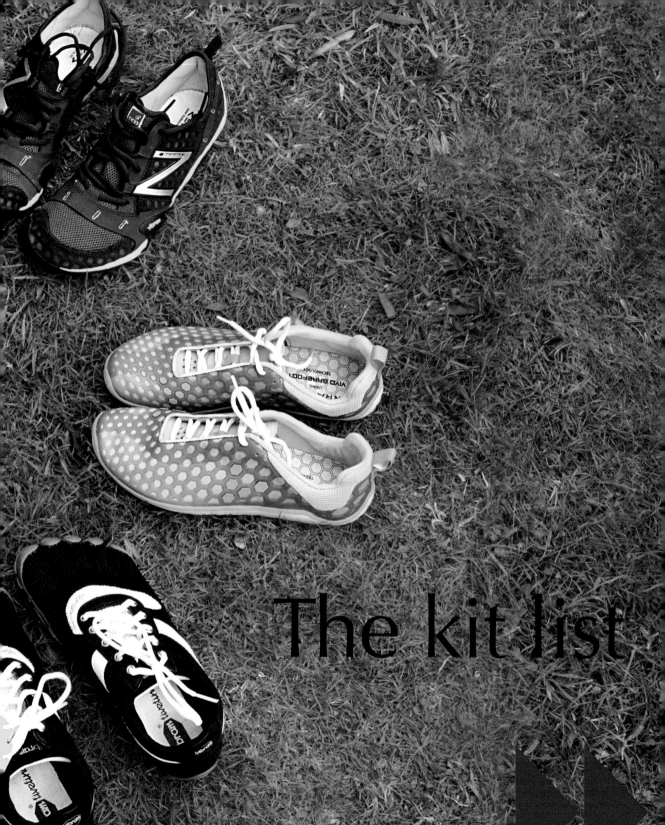

The kit list

Shoe shop

Choosing your most important piece of kit

Picking the right running shoes has never been easy, but in the past few years, the modern running shoe has undergone the greatest amount of change – and challenge – since its inception nearly five decades ago, rendering the decision even more bewildering.

After years of trainers being designed to 'control' movement and protect us from the ground with a thick layer of cushioning, there has been a definite shift towards a more minimalist approach. I'm talking about lighter, more flexible shoes with thinner midsoles and a smaller 'differential' (the difference between the height of the shoe at the heel and the forefoot). The trend has moved away from the 'bells and whistles' approach and towards shoes that leave the foot freer, promoting a more natural footstrike. This has been accompanied by a resurgence of interest in running technique and footstrike (see p. 46).

Why the change? Traditionally, the running shoe's major role has been to provide support and cushioning when you are moving forwards. The extent of each of these features can vary hugely and, in general, shoes with greater cushioning offer less stability and vice versa. The cushioning absorbs some of the landing force (twice to three times body weight), so you might think the more the better. But a growing body of research does not back this up. A study from the University of Virginia in 2009 found that in 68 adults (who ran at least 15 miles per week), joint forces were lower at the hip, knee and ankle when running barefoot. The theory is that lacking the tangibility of contact with a firm surface, the foot actually lands with greater force. Research from Harvard University in 2010 found that even on hard surfaces, barefoot runners generated smaller collision forces on impact than heel-striking shoe wearers.

Researchers speculate that runners adapt and modify their footstrike depending on the hardness of the surface or shoe. This is one of the arguments proposed by minimalist shoe and barefoot enthusiasts and it indicates that proprioception (awareness and 'feedback' from the ground) has a greater role to play in attenuating impact than was previously known. All of which makes a wedge of foam between your foot and the ground suddenly seem less desirable.

A thick layer of cushioning can also compromise flexibility. A shoe should bend at the metatarsophalangeal joint (the 'knuckle' of the foot). This is where your foot bends, so you don't want a shoe that prevents this or makes it difficult.

The other key role of the shoe, historically, has been to provide support – to guide your foot towards a 'neutral' gait which, it has always been believed, will leave you less injury prone. Some shoes (known as motion-control or stability shoes) have lots of support features to 'correct' your foot mechanics – for example, a medial post (an insert of plastic on the arch side, to give extra support) or a dual-density heel, on which the material on the medial side is harder than that on the lateral side, to prevent the foot from overpronating (see p. 49). Others (neutral or cushioned shoes) leave the foot more to its own devices.

In 2008, Dr Craig Richards, from the University of Newcastle in Australia, published a paper in the *British Journal of Sports Medicine* concluding that after extensive research, he couldn't find any evidence to show that running shoes made you less injury prone. He invited shoe manufacturers to respond if they held such evidence. None did, adding to the controversy.

While I'm quite a fan of the new minimalist running

shoes and even enjoy running barefoot sometimes, I think it's important not to throw the baby out with the bath water or disregard years of evolution in running shoe development.

Before modern running shoes, runners wore flat-soled pumps or plimsolls (not dissimilar to minimalist shoes) and didn't get injured. But running was not the mass participation sport it is today. In other words, there were far fewer people running who weren't 'naturals'. Nowadays, people of all ages and abilities run distances from 5km to a marathon and some do need some cushioning and support from their shoes, if only to make up for what they lack in technique. Without it, they may not be able to run problem-free.

I believe there is a place for both types of running shoe – from a featherweight super-minimalist racer to a solid stability trainer and everything in between. The question is, which pair is right for you?

Again, long-held wisdom on choosing running shoes has been challenged recently. It was once thought that if you had a high arch, you needed more cushioning, whereas flatter feet needed more support. But there are too many exceptions for such a systematic diagnosis to be acceptable any more, and studies looking at what feet do in motion have shown that it's possible to have a high arch and still overpronate like a flat-footer.

So where does all this leave you when you go shoe shopping? You'll find some guidance in my shoe shopping checklist over the page. Your types of run and the surfaces you run on will also inform your choice. There are shoes designed for running on rough terrain (trail or fell shoes), shoes for running fast (racing flats or, for the track, spikes) and shoes for high mileage. You may need more than one pair to meet all your needs. That's no bad thing as different shoes will demand a slight variation in your biomechanics, so you aren't continually stressing the same areas.

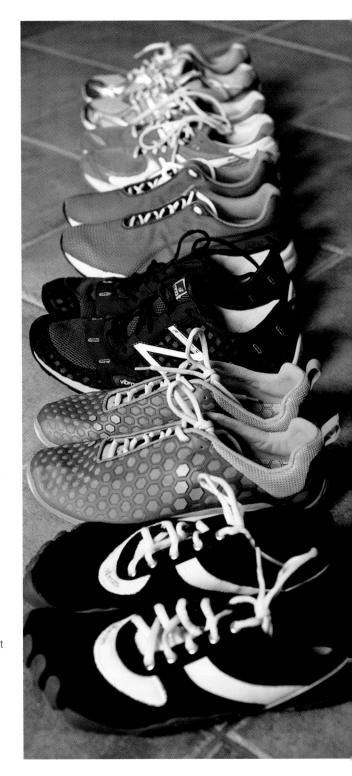

Shoe shopping checklist

- **Ask the experts** Go to a reputable, specialist running store with a good range of brands and models. Be prepared to answer lots of questions: what sort of surfaces do you run on? Have you had any injuries? They will want to look at your feet and, quite possibly, get you on a treadmill (or on the pavement) to assess your running in your current shoes and in any you are considering buying. If you don't receive this level of interest, go elsewhere.

- **Try it on** Try on lots of pairs before making a decision. Good fit is everything, and you shouldn't need to 'break in' running shoes. You need approximately an index finger's width beyond your longest toe to allow your foot to move. Don't worry if the size is bigger than for your normal shoes. I wear size 8 running shoes, which doesn't make me feel very ladylike (but nor did the black toenails I suffered when I opted for 7s). Don't just stand there looking at them in the mirror – you need to get a feel for how the shoes are to run in.

- **Be prepared** Remember to take the socks you normally run in. Take your old running shoes, if you have any. Go after a run, or towards the end of the day when your feet will have spread a little – this better reflects their shape and size during running. And stand, don't sit, when you're assessing the shoe.

- **Trust your instincts** Getting the right advice is important, but research suggests that your feet know what's best. One study found a high correlation between the shoe that felt 'right' to a runner and the shoe deemed to be right by gait analysis.

- **Less is more** While you may need some support or cushioning, I recommend opting for the 'least amount of shoe' that feels appropriate. Allowing your foot to move as naturally as possible is better than going for as much cushioning and/or stability as you can find.

- **If it ain't broke...** If you've already found a brand and model you like and are running comfortably and without injury, stick with them. Don't experiment just for the sake of it. If you do find your perfect shoe, buy more than one pair. Shoe manufacturers frequently change or discontinue models, and you'll be mourning them for ever more.

- **Be sport specific** Wear shoes designed for running, whether they are heavy-duty support shoes or minimalist trainers. A tennis shoe is designed for moving sideways as well as forwards and back, so it isn't stable enough for running, whereas a stiff-soled cross-trainer won't allow the foot to flex freely.

- **Pay the price** How much do you need to pay for decent shoes? You don't need to opt for the top-of-the-range models to get a good pair, but I would avoid the bottom end of the range and cheap shoes from non-specialist manufacturers, like supermarkets. Shop around – you can often find last season's model of a reputable shoe for a fraction of the original price.

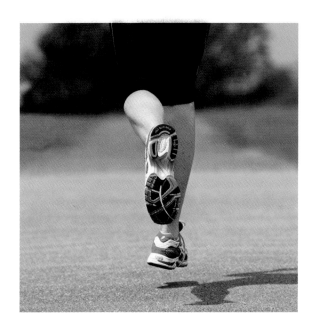

Do I need women-specific shoes?

A woman's foot typically has a greater difference between the width of the forefoot and rearfoot than a man's, and shoe manufacturers now offer most of their range in men's and women's fits, as well as female-specific models. You don't necessarily need a women's shoe. It's all about fit – if a man's shoe or model fits better, that's fine.

The lifespan of a running shoe

Running shoes generally last 300–500 miles, but looking after them will prolong their lifespan. Wear them only for running, and if they get wet or excessively sweaty, remove the insoles to air them and allow them to dry out. (If they get really wet, stuff newspaper inside them to absorb moisture and dry quicker.) It's great if you can have more than one pair, so the midsole can decompress between uses. Don't be tempted to throw them in the washing machine – use an old toothbrush and warm soapy water for cleaning and dry them away from artificial heat.

Sometimes it's obvious when a shoe has had its day, with frayed fabric or a trodden-down heel, but the signs are not always visible. The 'twist test' is a good indicator of whether a shoe has worn out. Hold it firmly at the heel and halfway along the forefoot and twist. If it gives easily, the midsole is no longer offering as much support and you could need a new pair. Press firmly down inside the shoe to check whether there is any cushioning left in the midsole. (These tests aren't relevant for minimal shoes, which don't have a firm, cushioned midsole.) I note in my training diary when I 'start' new shoes and what the model is called. Or you could write it under the insole in marker pen.

Tying the knot

The way you tie your laces can subtly alter the fit of a shoe. These three tying tricks can help common shoe-fit problems.

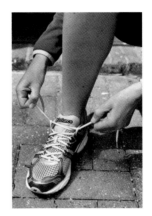

Heel slips around

Do a 'normal' criss-cross lacing pattern up to the penultimate hole. Then thread each end of the lace through the last hole on its own side, pulling a bit of lace up to create a loop. Take the end of each lace to the loop on the opposite side and pull tight.

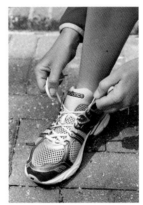

Shoe too wide

Use a criss-cross lacing pattern roughly halfway up the shoe. Then, as above, thread each end of the lace through the next hole on its own side, pulling a little bit of lace up to create a loop. Take the end of each lace to the loop on the opposite side and pull tight. Continue lacing to the end in a normal criss-cross.

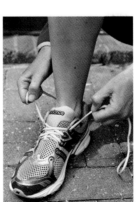

Shoe too narrow

Take the laces out completely and rethread them, starting from the third or fourth hole down, not from the far end.

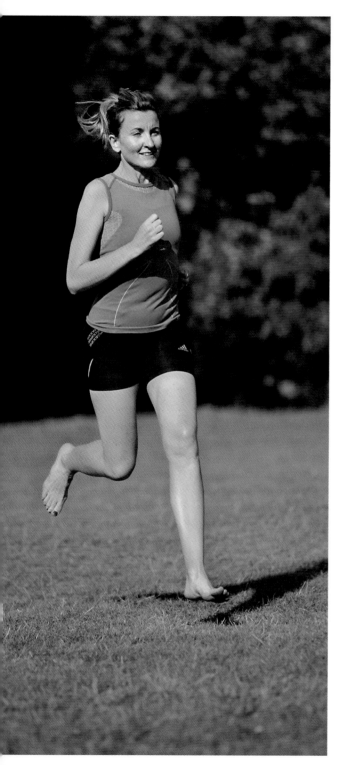

What about barefoot?

In *Run for Life*, I advised not running more than one mile barefoot, and building up to that slowly. Although I still recommend cautiously building up to unshod running, I now know that you can run a lot further because I've done it. I discovered the joys of barefoot running with John Woodward, an Alexander Technique teacher and running coach. I learned how much you can benefit from having direct contact with the ground, in terms of responsiveness and body awareness, as well as the pleasure of feeling the earth underneath your feet. One of the key things John taught me is that the foot is incredibly flexible, mobile and strong. Encased in shoes, we often think of our feet as slabs, which don't bend, stretch or flex – but they do, and wearing shoes that don't let them do this can leave them weak and stiff.

Although I don't run barefoot all the time, my experience has informed my choice of trainer, changing it quite considerably. I look for less weight, more flexibility, a smaller differential (or none at all) and a wide toe box to allow my toes to spread naturally.

To experiment with barefoot running, spend a few weeks walking barefoot at home and in the garden, and strengthen your foot muscles with exercises like heel and toe walking, spreading the toes as you step forwards, then scrunching them up to 'grab' the ground and practising moving your big toe and other toes independently. Then introduce some short strides – four reps of 50m at the end of your warm-up or run – and progress from there. Even if you limit your barefooting to a few strides or drills, you'll still be improving your foot strength and flexibility and enhancing technique.

Foot file

Being a runner doesn't mean you have to put up with horrible feet. Provided you take a little care, you should be able to bare your soles with pride.

It is a myth that you should 'harden up' your feet for running. Moisturise them regularly (any moisturiser will do) and use a pumice stone or foot file to smooth any hardened patches, particularly on the edge of the big toe and joint below it. A regular self-administered foot massage will boost circulation and soothe hard-working foot muscles. Cut toenails short and straight across. Here's how to deal with three common foot problems:

Athlete's foot

A fungal infection that appears as sore, cracked skin between the toes, athlete's foot thrives in damp, sweaty places.

Solution: use an over-the-counter anti-fungal product, such as Lamisil. Alternatively, try dabbing a cotton-wool ball moistened with water and a few drops of tea tree oil on affected areas. Consider replacing your trainer insoles or treat them with an anti-fungal in case the infection is harboured there.

Prevention: always dry thoroughly between your toes and wear flip-flops when walking barefoot on damp floors in public places, such as gym changing rooms.

Blisters

These are a result of friction between you and your footwear. It could be the seams of your socks, the fact that your shoe is slipping each time your foot strikes due to a poor fit, or an uneven surface, causing your foot to rub against the side of the shoe.

Solution: use a blister plaster, such as Compeed, to protect the area while the blister heals. If the fluid-filled area is causing discomfort, use a sterilised needle to pop it (pierce the blister in two places close to where it meets the skin).

Prevention: if you are very prone to blisters, use surgical tape to tape up the vulnerable areas and reassess your footwear – both shoes and socks. Recurring blisters, coupled with a build-up of hard skin on the joint below the big toe can indicate overpronation.

Bruised toenails

Black toenails are so common among runners they could be considered a rite of passage – but one best avoided. The problem usually affects the big toe (or second toe, if it is longer) and is caused by the toe rubbing against – or striking – the top of the shoe repeatedly, causing blood to pool beneath the nail.

Solution: if the toe is painless, leave the nail to fall off by itself, but apply an anti-fungal cream to prevent infection. If the toe is throbbing and painful, your doctor or podiatrist will need to make a hole in the nail to relieve the pressure and drain the blood.

Prevention: ensure that your shoes have plenty of room in the toe box. Keep your nails well trimmed. The lacing technique shown on p. 119 will help keep your heel snugly in place, preventing the foot slipping forwards.

What to wear
Choosing the right kit

You can run in any lightweight, comfortable clothing. Just avoid garments so flappy you might trip over them or so tight they chafe or restrict your movement. So why pay for running-specific kit? The key differences are in the fabric and cut.

Clever clobber

Running kit maximises streamlining, allowing freedom of movement without excess fabric. You don't have to don skin-tight tops and Lycra shorts – it could be a pair of loose-cut pants with a zip-up long-sleeved top. Running gear has other useful features, like pockets for your keys, thumbholes in sleeves to anchor the top over your hands and save you wearing gloves, air vents to aid breathability and flat seams to minimise chafing.

All high-tech materials are breathable, so you don't overheat, and sweat-wicking, drawing moisture away from the skin, ensuring you don't get too sweaty or rubbed up the wrong way. They are lightweight, so you aren't carrying around extra weight – imagine how heavy a pair of rain-drenched sweatpants could get. Some specialist materials, like Windstopper or Paclite, protect you from the wind and rain, while others, like Polartec, are thermal to conserve body heat or have built-in sun protection.

Reflectivity and visibility are also important. There are two different measurements of visibility: 'perception distance', the point at which a driver has spotted something and 'recognition distance', the point at which they've recognised the 'something' as a runner. Even in daylight, wearing fluorescent clothing will improve perception distance. If you're running after dark, you need to go further because while fluorescent clothes will improve perception distance significantly, reflective

materials and lights can increase recognition distance to as much as 200m. Movement aids recognition in poor visibility, so look for garments with reflective strips on 'moving parts', the arms and legs, to make yourself easier to spot.

In all but the warmest conditions, layering is the best way to dress, trapping air between layers, increasing warmth and allowing you to remove or add garments to regulate body temperature. But for layering to work efficiently, all your clothing needs to be breathable and sweat-wicking – otherwise, moisture will get trapped.

Support strategy

One running-specific item you can't do without is a sports bra. That's true whether you are a 32AA or a 38G. The breasts move in a figure-of-eight pattern when we run, and research demonstrates that even an A-cup breast moves 4.2cm away from the body, stretching the Cooper's ligaments (thin bands of fibrous, non-elastic tissue that cover and support the breasts). If the breasts are poorly supported, then over time these ligaments will stretch irreversibly, causing your boobs to sag. Poorly supported could mean not bothering with a sports bra at all, or it could mean wearing the wrong size or type. The *Journal of Science and Medicine in Sport* found that 85 per cent of women were not wearing the right bra size when exercising – causing pain and discomfort – even putting some women off physical activity completely.

There are encapsulated bras, in which each breast is supported within its own cup, sometimes with underwiring, and compression bras, which control movement by pressing the breasts against the rib cage. Women with larger breasts used to be advised to opt for encapsulated bras and smaller-chested women for compression types, but a 2009 study from the University of Portsmouth found that encapsulated styles offered all women greater support.

You'll need to try on a few bras before deciding on the right one. This doesn't rule out mail order (companies like Lessbounce.com often have a far greater range than shops), as you can return unwanted items. The best way of finding your correct size is to be measured by a professional. Make sure your bra ticks these boxes:

- It should fit snugly without restricting your breathing.
- You should be able to slide one finger under the strap – if you can fit more fingers, it isn't tight enough.
- The shoulder straps and back clasp should be adjustable, so you can achieve a perfect fit (and tighten when it 'gives' with use). Choose a bra which doesn't require you to use the tightest clasp when it's new to achieve the right fit.
- The strap should sit horizontally all the way round, rather than riding up at the back.
- The straps should be wide enough not to dig into your skin, and seams should not chafe.
- Monthly hormonal fluctuations can influence breast size, so you may need two different sizes.

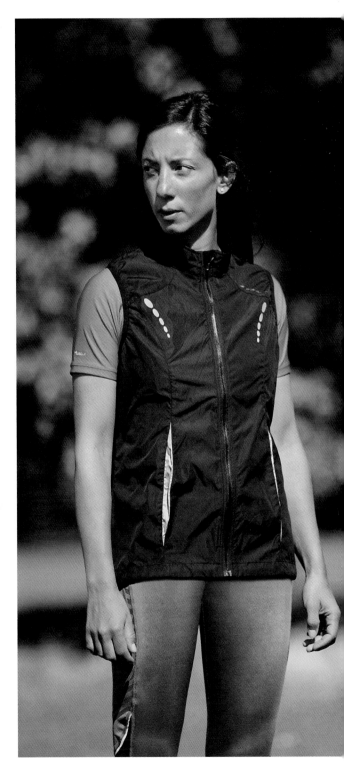

> Don't let being a big-boobed runner hold you back. As a size 34E, finding the right sports bra (in my case, the Enell) changed my life. When I run now, nothing bounces.
>
> Fiona

Your running wardrobe

These are the essentials for my 'capsule' running wardrobe (season-specific gear is covered in 'Winter Running' opposite and 'Summer Survival' on p.126.)

- Short- and long-sleeved technical tops (and a couple of vests, which I mainly use for racing).
- Shorts or capri-length tights – different degrees of coverage; shorts include traditional, loose-running shorts as well as Lycra bike-style shorts.
- A 'base layer' – a thin garment designed to be worn next to the skin; in cooler climes it forms the basis of your layering.
- Full-length tights or loose pants – not just for winter running (I often wear full tights when running on rough off-road routes to protect myself from nettles and ticks).
- Water-resistant jacket – an all-year round essential. Strike a balance between breathability and water-resistance depending on typical climate. Removable sleeves are a great asset for added versatility.
- Running socks – from knee-high compression socks to thin trainer liners and padded anklets (see Sock shop).
- Compression tights – read more on p. 126.

Buying proper running gear is so worthwhile once you are going regularly. My first pair of running tights was a revelation after leggings that rode up or fell down.

Sarah T

Sock shop

When you start running, you might wear any old pair, but once you've discovered the joys of decent running socks, you'll never go back. What joys? An absence of seams, or flat-stitched seams that don't chafe, double-layer socks for blister prevention, sweat-wicking and anti-fungal fabrics like X-static, which is designed to prevent socks from getting smelly and reduce the risk of infection.

Running socks are usually 'shaped' too, which stops them bunching up. Knee-high compression socks (see p. 126) are another option. If you're constantly hampered by blisters, don't even think about wearing bog-standard cotton sports socks. Although they absorb moisture superbly, they aren't able to do anything with it, causing the fabric to swell and create friction. In a US study comparing technical fabric socks to cotton ones, runners found that the cotton socks lost their shape and wrinkled up – perfect conditions for blisters. Technical fibres performed much better and kept the runners' feet drier, which is good news when you consider that the average foot can sweat over 500ml a day. Find running socks at your specialist running store or adventure travel shop.

Winter running

As the saying goes, 'There's no such thing as bad weather, only inappropriate clothing!' If it's already raining when you set off, you should be kitted out in a breathable waterproof jacket. If it looks like rain, you might want to consider wearing a jacket, or tying it around your waist. If you are driving somewhere to run, carry a towel and dry clothing in the car, so that you don't have to sit around in wet clothing afterwards.

Your extremities are most at risk in cold weather, as blood is shunted to more vital areas such as your internal organs, as well as blood vessels near to the skin surface close to prevent heat loss. Here are some winter warmers to consider:

- **Thermals** A thermal base layer and thermal tights offer extra protection against the cold.
- **Gloves** (or mittens, which are better, although a bit restrictive) In less Baltic conditions, tops with hook-over thumbholes can be useful to keep the hands warm until you start to generate some heat.
- **Hat** A beanie or similar will keep your ears warm. It's also useful for tucking your hair into and making your gender less obvious.
- **Waterproof socks** If you are running on wet ground and your trainers are going to get soaked, waterproof socks are a godsend (see Resources, p. 204).

Follow the tips below if you are running on a cold day:

- Warm up for longer.
- Eat before you run – you'll need to insulate yourself against the cold.
- Don't forgo hydration. You may not feel as if you are sweating, but once you're on the move, you will be.
- Don't go so far that you run out of energy and have to walk back or slow down considerably. Your body will cool down really quickly and leave you shivering.
- Watch your footing in icy conditions.
- Avoid speed work with long recoveries in which you will quickly cool down.

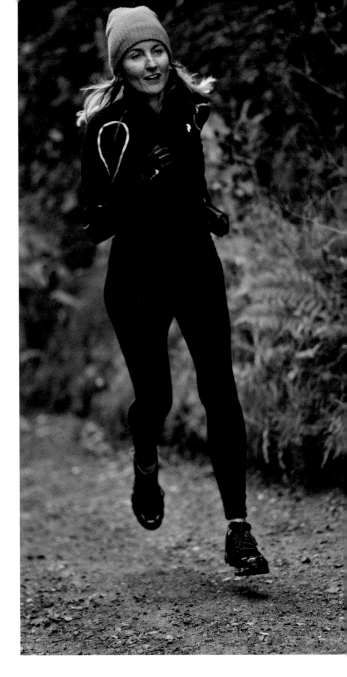

- If you suffer from asthma, cold weather may aggravate it. This is one instance where breathing through your nose instead of your mouth can help. Or begin running with a scarf or antipollution mask over your face to 'warm' the air before it reaches your airways. And always warm up slowly and thoroughly.

Take care of your running kit

- Non-biological washing detergents are best; there are even specific sports wash formulas, which will prolong the life of your technical fabrics and prevent odour.
- Follow directions on labels, like doing up zips and washing inside out.
- Don't leave kit lying around sweaty or damp – it will wear out much quicker.

Summer survival

If you live, or are visiting, somewhere hot and humid, you'll need to take extra precautions regarding fluid intake and clothing to avoid overheating.

- Wear lightweight, breathable kit – a vest is cooler than a T-shirt, allowing more air to circulate.
- Carry fluids with you, even on shorter runs (you sweat more in hot conditions so need to drink more than usual).
- Protect yourself with sunglasses. Sport sunglasses are designed to stay on even when you are moving around, and usually have a wraparound style and a sweat-resistant nose bridge to prevent slippage. They also protect you from dust and flies.
- Consider wearing a hat or visor; a baseball hat works fine, but a visor prevents your head getting hot, while keeping the sun off your face.
- Use sunscreen, even if it is overcast. You need one that's at least factor 15 and filters out both UVA and UVB rays. Choose a sport-specific formula that will stay on even when you sweat. I'm a big fan of once-a-day silicone-based formulas.
- Bear in mind that running in the heat will slow you down. Run when the day is cooler and less humid.

The latest squeeze: compression gear

Compression clothing – including socks, tights and tops – is designed to improve your performance and enhance recovery. The theory is that by holding muscles tightly, oscillation (wobbling) is reduced, leading to less muscle damage. It's also claimed that they promote circulation and the return of blood to the heart. Research has been equivocal (a 2010 study from Indiana University concluded that compression clothing had no significant effect on performance), but in some cases, even when a measurable performance benefit wasn't found, the participants still perceived their performance to be better. One area in which the results seem promising is in recovery. Research from Ball State University, Indiana, found that using compression gear following maximal exertion prevented loss of range of motion, reduced swelling and promoted the recovery of force production. Another study, in the *Journal of Sports Science and Medicine*, showed that wearing graduated compression tights (in which the compression is greatest at the ankle and diminishes further up the leg) after a period of strenuous downhill walking hastened recovery by allowing faster cell repair. Again, there may be a psychological element – I look forward to putting on a pair of compression tights post-run as I feel it takes some of the stress off my muscles and it simply feels good. (See Resources, p. 204, for suppliers.)

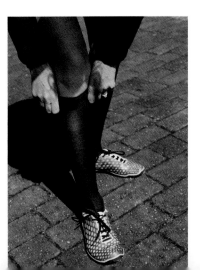

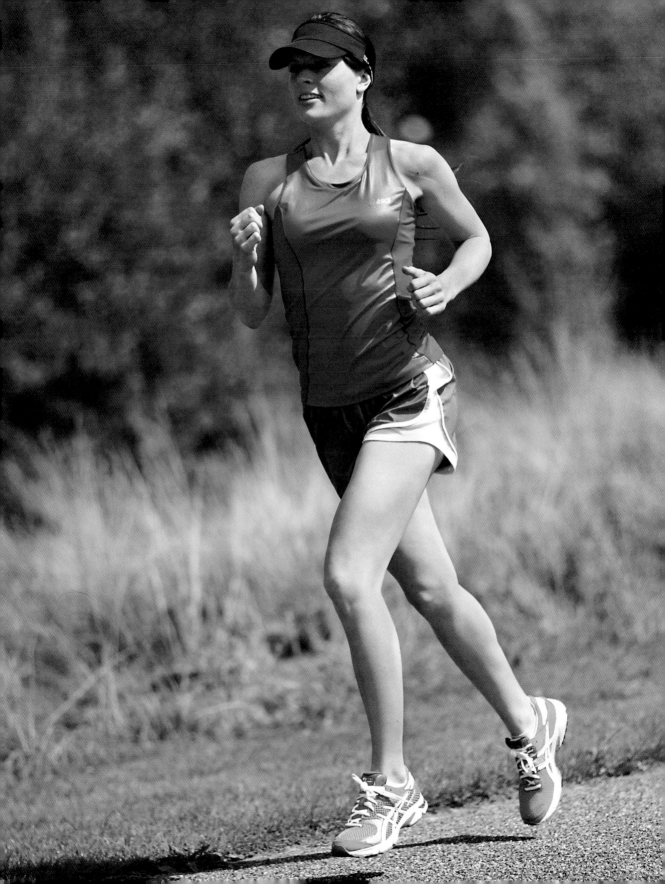

Carry the load

Whether it's a rucksack big enough for all your work gear or a hip belt to carry a few essentials, make sure you choose a bag specifically designed for running. That way, it won't jiggle up and down as you run, nor will the straps dig in or chafe.

Many companies make female-specific rucksacks, with shoulder straps placed closer together for a better fit. I've found that rucksacks with lots of different compartments work best, as the contents don't move around as much, and it's easier to locate items. The other key thing is to have adjustable straps both at the waist and across the chest to keep the pack snug and secure. Many rucksacks have space for a hydration pack with a feed tube that comes over the shoulder and gives you an on-tap supply of fluid. Some bags are designed specifically for carrying fluid, although most will have space for carrying other items.

Hip belts are good if you just want to carry a couple of bottles or gels. Look for an adjustable belt that stays put and doesn't chafe or ride up. See Resources, p. 205.

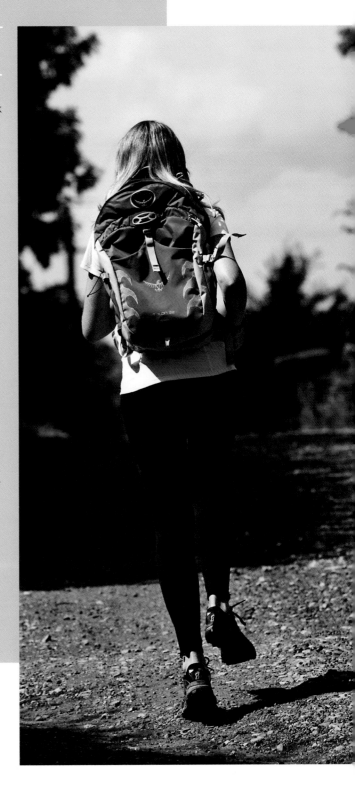

Training tools
Gadgets for monitoring performance

Running is often lauded for its simplicity, but there's a world of gadgets available, promising to monitor, record and even enhance your performance. None is essential, but heart-rate monitors, GPS watches and the like can be very useful. Their biggest advantage is giving real-time feedback on everything from your minutes-per-mile pace, to distance covered, heart rate and calorie expenditure (and that's just the basics). Why is such data useful?

Well, while you are running it can really help to have a feel for different paces or effort levels – (this is what a 7.30-minute mile feels like – could I keep this up for the whole 5km race...?) From a longer-term perspective, there's a lot to be gained from reviewing your runs. Even if you don't want to spend hours analysing data, storing information from your runs, on the gadget itself, or by downloading it on to your computer, gives you the bigger picture on how your training is going, and might reveal aspects you could change. You might notice that you run better in the morning, so alter when you schedule tougher sessions; or you might see that your heart rate on a tempo run has dropped, and push the pace a little more next time. Run feedback can also act as a pat on the back – it's very motivating to see your pace increase as you get fitter.

These devices take into account your personal statistics, like age, gender, weight, height and training status, increasing their accuracy and making their data more meaningful. But I do think there's a tendency to rely too heavily on gadgets, particularly GPS watches. It's important to hone your 'feel' for running so that you can listen to your body when gauging your effort. Use it wisely, but don't let gadgetry take over from instinct.

The three most useful parameters to monitor are your pace, distance and your heart rate.

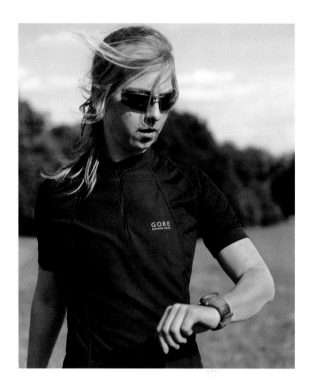

"

Get to know the staff at your local running shop. You'll get a far more personal service that way and they can help out with recommendations for races, physios, etc.

Sue

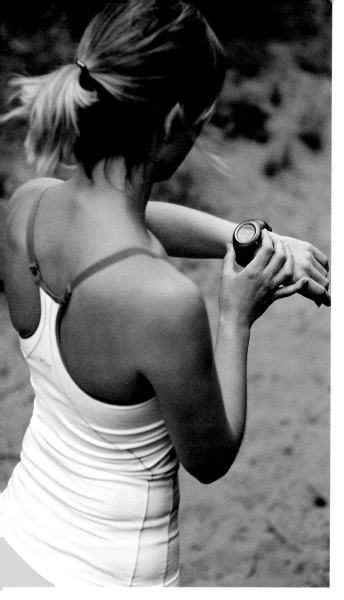

performance. You can even use it to race your 'virtual self' on a regular route. You can download sessions to your computer, which will store and/or compare to previous runs, generating even more information (such as where the hills were or a map of your route). On the downside, you can only use GPS outdoors (not much use if you run on the treadmill), and, depending on the quality of the receiver, the signal can be lost in very built-up areas, under heavy tree cover or on a twisting run. The issue of GPS devices being heavy is slowly being solved, but there is still a problem with short battery life and the need for regular recharging. See Resources, p. 204.

Speed–distance devices

Another option for measuring your pace is a speed–distance monitor. At the basic end of the spectrum is a pedometer, which uses your stride length (which you tell it) and number of strides you take (which it 'counts' via the movement of your hip) to estimate distance travelled. These are mostly used for walking and tend not to be very accurate for running because they cannot account for your stride lengthening or shortening in response to different paces or terrain. Top-end speed–distance monitors are far more sophisticated and almost as accurate as GPS. They use motion sensors called accelerometers which are located within a foot pod, worn in or on the shoe. These sensors measure acceleration more than 1000 times per second, using complex algorithms to calculate speed and distance. There's no need to measure your stride length, but most models do give you the option to calibrate (by timing yourself running a measured distance), to enhance accuracy. Another useful feature, which a GPS watch cannot offer, is cadence monitoring, i.e. counting the number of steps you take per minute. Speed–distance devices can be used indoors (e.g. on a treadmill) and don't rely on an external signal that could be interrupted. Battery life is generally much longer than GPS devices too, but the price difference between the two isn't as great as you would expect.

GPS

A GPS device is usually a watch, but could also come via your phone or other hand-held device. The biggest plus is that GPS offers accurate satellite-derived information on your speed, pace per mile or kilometre, location and distance covered. I use my GPS watch for all sessions in which I desire to run at a specific pace (e.g. a threshold run or interval session). Many GPS devices come with (or offer, as an additional purchase) a chest strap for heart-rate monitoring, enabling you to track every aspect of

Heart-rate monitors

The more effort you put into a run, the more times per minute your heart has to beat in order to pump sufficient blood to the working muscles. A heart rate monitor (HRM) measures not how fast you are going but how hard you are working. In some situations, that can be a good thing. If you are running on undulating terrain, your pace will fluctuate greatly, but it doesn't mean you are slacking off. If you are running after a particularly tiring day or in hot, humid conditions, your pace may be slower than usual, although you're working just as hard. If you were measuring only your pace, you might beat yourself up about that, but monitoring heart rate demonstrates that your cardiovascular system is as taxed as usual.

By providing an up-to-the-minute snapshot of your effort level, an HRM can tell you what kind of 'training effect' you're getting, regardless of your pace, activity, terrain or conditions, so it could be considered more forgiving than the GPS system that simply tells you: 'Not achieving those eight-minute miles today.'

An HRM consists of a chest strap and a watch. It transmits heart-rate data in real time, as well as recording averages to display after the run. If you've read about the importance of working at a range of different intensities (see Chapter 4), you'll realise why having a method of monitoring your effort is so useful. Most HRMs allow you to input your personal data (age, gender, activity level, etc.) and will then set upper and lower thresholds – some will bleep if you go outside these. I prefer models that allow you to adjust them manually.

Heart-rate monitoring isn't good for runs consisting of short bouts of effort, as there is a delay between you beginning to run fast and your heart rate increasing in response. It can take between 60 and 120 seconds for heart rate to respond and achieve a steady state during short, intense efforts. If you were running intervals of three to four minutes, heart-rate readings may not be accurate for a big chunk of each interval.

Running apps

There are countless running apps to help you plot, monitor and record your run – some use your phone's in-built GPS to track your route, pace and distance, while others enable you to pre-set pace or distance, and give you feedback and encouragement via headphones as you run. More sophisticated apps enable you to store, analyse, compare and share run data on your phone, but one of my favourites is the simplest, which acts as a metronome, helping me improve my cadence by giving me a rhythm to move my feet to.

One thing heart-rate monitoring is very good for is for reining you in on easy runs. Many of us run our easy runs too hard and our hard runs too easy. By setting the upper limits of your easy run in heart-rate terms, you can ensure you don't overdo it.

Like GPS, many HRMs enable you to download and store data on your computer. But don't spend money on functions you won't use. More expensive models will have a better 'sampling' rate, meaning they collect heart-rate data more frequently, making them more accurate. Ensure that the monitor is easy to set up and use, otherwise it'll end up at the bottom of your kit bag.

All sounding like too much information? If all you really want to know is how long you have been running for, a simple sports watch will do the job just fine. Plenty of runners are happy with nothing more technical than a cheap digital watch. Useful features include a countdown timer for interval training, a 'split time' function to record lap times, a screen that lights up for running in the dark and accessible buttons.

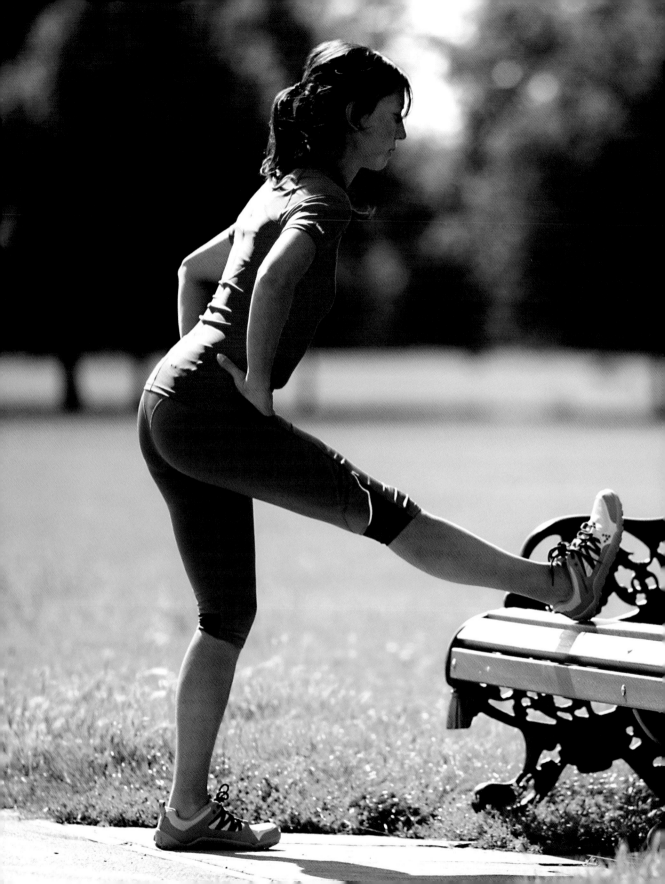

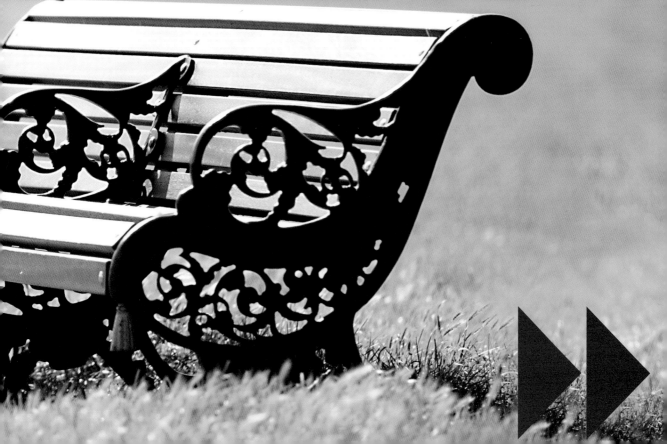

Food and drink

Fuel for thought

There's no magic ingredient in the runner's diet. Like any healthy diet, it should offer a good balance of the three major nutrients: carbohydrate, protein and fat, with plenty of fresh fruit and vegetables, and wholegrains.

But there are two ways in which the runner's diet should be different. The first is the overall amount of energy – the second, timing. Running burns calories – lots of 'em. So runners need more calories daily to sustain their body weight. A calorie is the unit used to measure how much energy is provided by what we eat and drink.

Although all major nutrients provide calories, their contribution varies; for example, 1 gram of fat provides 9 calories while 1 gram of protein provides just 4. To complicate matters, foods are rarely made up of one type of nutrient (e.g. 100 per cent fat). They tend to contain a mixture of protein and fat, or carbohydrate and protein, and their total energy content will be the sum of the calories provided by each component. That's why the art of reading food labels is a useful one to master.

But knowing how many calories are in a food is only meaningful if you know how many calories you should be consuming. To find out you'll have to get your head around a few terms first.

All about energy

Our 'total daily energy expenditure' (TDEE) is made up of 'basal metabolic rate' (BMR, the amount of energy we need to exist) and 'physical activity level' (PAL, our daily exercise and activity level).

To estimate your daily calorie requirement, complete the following calculations:

1. Calculate your weight in kilograms
2. Put your weight into the relevant formula to get a basal metabolic rate (BMR):

- 10–18 years old: weight x 12.2; answer + 746 = BMR
- 18–30 years old: weight x 14.7; answer + 496 = BMR
- 31–60 years old: weight x 8.7; answer + 829 = BMR
- 60+ years old. Weight x 10.5; answer + 596 = BMR

3. Multiply your BMR figure by the 'PAL' number that most closely matches the amount of exercise (including running) you do.

- Mostly inactive – multiply BMR by 1.2
- Exercise 1–2 times per week – multiply BMR by 1.3
- Exercise 2–3 times per week – multiply BMR by 1.4
- Exercise 4–5 times per week – multiply BMR by 1.5
- Exercise 6–7 days per week – multiply BMR by 1.7

The answer is an approximation of how much energy you typically burn in a day (TDEE). Consuming this number of calories will maintain your weight. If you want to shed or gain weight, that's another matter! (See p. 140 for more information on running and weight.)

How many calories does running burn?

The average expenditure is approximately 100 calories per mile. Surprisingly, there isn't that much difference in the calories expended in running a mile fast or slow. If you want a more accurate estimate of your calories-per-mile rate use the following formula:

1 calorie per kilogram of body weight, per kilometre run (on the flat).

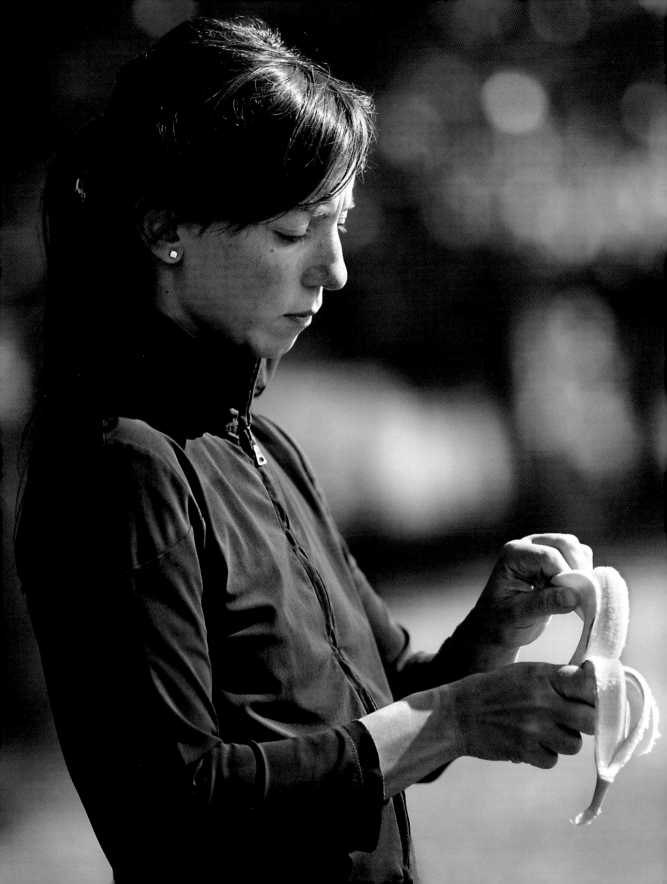

What to eat

If we were just concerned with our overall calorie consumption, it wouldn't matter whether we got our calories from 25 bananas or six chocolate bars, but foods also provide other nutrients – vitamins, minerals, amino acids, phytochemicals – that have a huge impact on our health, not to mention our ability to run well, so we need to get the balance right.

Carbohydrates

Runners are always talking about 'carbs', or carbohydrates – and for good reason. Carbohydrate is the body's preferred energy source for physical activity. It is converted into glycogen, which is stored in the muscles and liver, and glucose, transported by the blood. It's the only fuel the brain can use, so if there isn't sufficient carbohydrate present, alternative fuel sources need to be converted into glucose.

The body has an infinite capacity for storing fat – but the same does not hold true for carbohydrate. We only store enough carbohydrate to fuel 90–120 minutes of strenuous exercise like running – so it needs to feature regularly in the runner's diet.

Since runners expend more energy on exercise than sedentary people, they need more than the typical carbohydrate intake of 40 to 50 per cent of total calories. Nutritionists recommend working out your needs based on your body weight, rather than using a percentage of energy intake. Guidelines vary, but approximately 4–7g per kilogram of body weight is a good aim for recreational to serious runners (the more you run, the more you'll need).

How much carbohydrate?

The carbohydrate content of some common foods

1 medium bowl (40g) porridge made with 200ml semi-skimmed milk 34g

1 medium banana 34.8g

1 teaspoon honey 13g

6 dried apricots 25g

1 large jacket potato 80g

1 slice malt loaf 20.6g

1 medium portion (75g uncooked weight) brown basmati rice 54g

1 slice wholemeal bread 13.5g

1 large white pitta bread 43g

1 standard tin baked beans (207g) 45g

240g (cooked weight) spaghetti 66g

200ml semi skimmed milk 20g

2 Weetabix 25.7g

40g (medium) serving All Bran 20g

1 wholewheat tortilla 16.2g

1 cereal bar (30g) 19g

1 bottle Gatorade 30g

GI IQ

The 'glycaemic index' (GI) is a measure of how quickly a carbohydrate releases sugar into the bloodstream. The calculation is based on the amount of a foodstuff required to provide 50g carbohydrate. For good health, the advice is to stick to low- to moderate-GI foods (such as brown basmati rice, lentils, wholegrain bread, wholewheat pasta, oats, beans and pulses, and unpeeled new potatoes) and to steer clear of high-GI foods (such as white bread and pasta, mashed potato, tropical fruits, refined-sugar products like jam, sugary drinks, dried fruits). This is because high-GI foods generally cause blood sugar levels to rise sharply and then drop, rather than providing a sustained energy release. This can cause energy highs and lows, and may have you reaching for a quick-fix snack. But there are a few caveats for runners.

Firstly, research from the University of Sydney suggests that physically active people don't experience the same peak in blood sugar as a result of eating high-GI foods, so need worry about it less. Secondly, there are times when high-GI foods are positively useful. If you want to go running before work and don't have time to digest a low-GI bowl of porridge, you could choose half a bagel with jam instead. Need energy on the run? Drink an isotonic sports drink.

Although GI can be helpful in making dietary choices, it can be misleading. Carrots and watermelon have a GI of over 70, making them high-GI. This might lead you to assume that they are off-limits. But given that a slice of watermelon only contains 5.6g of carbohydrate (it's mostly water), you'd need to eat huge amounts to experience a blood sugar spike. This holds true for nearly all fruits and vegetables. That's where the glycaemic load (GL) comes in.

While still measuring the blood sugar response of carbohydrates, GL takes into account the amount of carbohydrate there is in a typical serving of the food, rather than a fixed 50g amount. In the context of GL, carrots and watermelon classify as 'low'.

A final factor to bear in mind is that we tend not to eat foods in isolation. The presence of other nutrients, such as protein and fat, can attenuate the blood sugar response to a high-GI carbohydrate. Mashed potato eaten with salmon and leafy green vegetables will not trigger the same response as mashed potato on its own.

Consider GI and GL when selecting carbohydrates, but don't base every decision on them. Stick to unrefined and wholegrain products where possible, but don't be afraid to use high-GI foodstuffs for an instant energy boost before or during running or to hasten recovery.

Do I need to carbo-load?

In general training, there is no need to obsess over carbohydrates. If you are meeting the guidelines outlined, then you are doing fine. The only time carbo-loading might be valuable is in the days before a marathon or other ultra-long duration event (if a half marathon takes you longer than two and a half hours, additional carbohydrate may be of use). The strategy used to be to deprive yourself of carbohydrates for three to four days, about a week before the race, then follow with an intensive two- to three-day period of cramming in loads – the theory being that your glycogen stores would absorb more in response to the prior shortage. Nowadays, the advice is simply to up your intake for the three to seven days before the race. Make sure it is extra carbs that you're eating and not extra food!

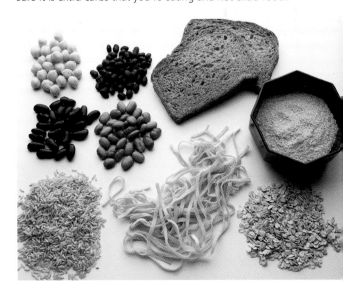

Protein

Protein doesn't play a major role in supplying energy for running (although in the absence of sufficient carbohydrate, it can be broken down to yield energy), but it is a vital nutrient in muscle tissue maintenance and repair – aiding recovery from and adaptation to running. Protein has a role in replacing oxygen-carrying red blood cells and supporting the immune system too. That's why you need a little more protein than a non-runner. The American College of Sports Medicine recommends 1.2–1.4g per kilogram of body weight per day for active people – compared to 0.8g for sedentary people. This should equate to around 15–18 per cent of your total energy intake. If you are new to running, be particularly vigilant about getting enough; research shows that in the early days of exercise, the body is less efficient at conserving and recycling protein. But don't think that if some is good, more must be better. Excess protein won't increase muscle growth or improve recovery, and if it's not needed for energy, it will be stored as fat.

Fat

The average woman has enough fat stored to fuel around 1200 miles (2000 km) of running, but the body prefers to use its less-abundant carbohydrate stores as a fuel source. While one of the most gratifying effects of training is that it enhances your capacity to use fat as a fuel, that isn't a green card to eat more. Most of us already consume more fat than we need. While research shows that more people now meet the UK government's recommendation of a fat intake of no more than 35 per cent of overall calorie intake, over half the population remains overweight or obese. Either we are consuming too many calories from other sources and exceeding our recommended daily energy intake, or the 35 per cent guideline is too high. I believe that both are true, but the latter is perhaps more relevant to runners. Why? Firstly, because runners need a slightly higher amount of carbohydrate and protein than non-runners, leaving less 'room' in the diet for fat; and secondly, because running involves carrying your body

weight, so excess weight will slow you down and increase the impact forces on your joints. I suggest aiming for 25–30 per cent of your overall energy intake from fat. If you consume 2000 calories per day, that means 500–600 calories can come from fat. Since 1g fat = 9 calories, that means 55–67g of fat per day. Many foods state fat grams on their label, so get into the habit of checking.

How much protein?

The protein content of some common foods

1 tin (200g) tuna in brine 47g

1 x 40g piece Cheddar cheese, grated 10g

½ standard tin of kidney beans 8.7g

200ml chocolate Nesquik made with
semi-skimmed milk 7.4g

1 chicken breast (125g) 30g

1 salmon fillet (150g) 30g

1 tin sardines in brine (120g) 19.5g

1 rounded teaspoon (15g) peanut butter 3.75g

1 tin (415g) baked beans 19g

1 small lean fillet steak (105g) 31g

200ml semi-skimmed milk 5.6g

25g mixed seeds 7g

1 carton (150g) natural yogurt 6g

1 medium egg 8g

Good fats, bad fats

While all types of fat contain the same number of calories, gram for gram, they differ significantly in their effect on our health. The best sources of fat are monounsaturated sources, like olive oil and rapeseed oil, avocados and seeds, and omega-3 fatty acids, which are a type of polyunsaturated fat derived primarily from oily fish, like salmon and mackerel, but also from walnuts and flaxseed. Omega-6 fatty acids, another type of polyunsaturated fat (found in sunflower oil and vegetable oil, and foods made with them) are also important in the diet, but most people eat more omega-6 than omega-3, when the ratio should be reversed. The fats to cut down on are saturated fats which come from meat and dairy products and processed foods like pies, biscuits and cakes. Try to avoid trans fats wherever possible. Like saturated fats, trans fats encourage the body to produce more 'bad' LDL cholesterol but they also lower 'good' HDL cholesterol – the perfect formula for heart disease. Trans fats are scarce in nature – they are created by turning a liquid fat (vegetable oil) into a solid fat – and are found mostly in highly processed foods, including manufactured cakes and pastries, low-fat spreads and commercial fried foods. Many manufacturers are eliminating trans fats from their products, so do check labels.

Perfect timing

Getting the timing of what we eat right is important for fuelling runs and facilitating recovery. In a nutshell, the rule is carbohydrates before exercise (and during, where necessary) and protein afterwards.

Before a run

Glycogen or carbohydrate is your five-star fuel. You need to keep glycogen stores topped up in order not to run out of energy. But what if you haven't had time to eat? For an easy or steady run, you can get away with eating on your return. But if it's a tough session or a long run, eat something an hour or two before. This is where high-GI foods are useful. A slice of malt loaf, a sports drink or a

few jelly babies within the hour before your run should do the trick. If you run after work, split your lunch into two, eating the second half mid-afternoon to avoid a long 'fast' after your last meal. If you simply can't eat beforehand, use a sports drink during tougher sessions.

You could choose to 'run on empty'. Some coaches advocate this, claiming that it burns more fat than fuelling up first. There is some truth to this, but that doesn't make it a good strategy. Running on an empty stomach can cause low blood sugar (hypoglycaemia), which could leave you feeling tired, dizzy and lightheaded, and will increase your 'perception of effort'. You're less likely to run as far, or as fast, as you would if you'd fuelled up first. It also risks you overcompensating when you return feeling ravenous. In my opinion, you'll get more out of your session if you don't run in a depleted energy state.

On the run

If you're just pootling around the block, there's no need to consume calories during your run. Even runs of 60–75 minutes can be done without topping up energy levels (especially if you are trying to lose weight). But when you're running for longer, some easily accessible carbohydrate will help to maintain blood sugar levels: research shows that consuming carbohydrate on long runs helps you to go further and faster, compared to drinking water. Your carb supply is most likely to be in the form of a sports drink or energy gel. You could choose to eat food instead, but it's trickier to get the amounts right and there's a greater risk of upsetting your stomach. Aim to take on 25–60g carbohydrate per hour – the equivalent of 400ml–1 litre of sports drink, 1–3 energy gels or 5–12 jelly babies. I recommend starting at the lower end of the range and seeing how you go.

Refuelling and recovery

If you have done a particularly long or hard run, a carbohydrate-based snack can help to restock glycogen stores, which will be depleted. There is a 'window of opportunity' in the first half hour post-run, when glycogen stores are particularly receptive, but this is not the only chance to restore glycogen; given time, the body will replenish depleted energy stores of its own accord.

You need to consider whether you need a post-run snack or if you should simply wait until your next mealtime (remembering to rehydrate). If you're trying to shed or maintain weight, a snack could represent excess calories. Ask yourself these questions to determine whether to carb up or wait up:

- Have I done a long run (60 minutes plus)?
- Was it a particularly demanding session?
- Will I be running again tomorrow?

If the answer to at least two of these is 'Yes', then aim to eat 1g carbohydrate for every kilogram of your body weight to optimise refuelling (or go for 50g as a ballpark figure). Always replace carbohydrate for any run longer than 90 minutes, regardless of intensity and training schedule.

The other important nutrient post-run is protein, owing to its vital role in repair and recovery. Research shows that consuming some protein with your carbs optimises recovery. The 'ideal' ratio is 3:1 (carbohydrate to protein) and there are many sports bars and drinks that fit the bill. But there's no reason why you can't achieve the right balance from food – a cheese or tuna sandwich, a bagel with peanut butter or a flavoured milk drink.

Running for weight loss

Many women start running to lose weight. It's a smart choice – running burns more calories per minute than most other endurance activities (combining it with strength training is even better – research shows that this helps to protect lean muscle mass, so you lose fat, not muscle). For best results, increasing calorie burning through exercise should be coupled with reducing calorie intake through diet. That way, you're tackling both ends of the equation.

There's a fine balance to be struck between eating fewer calories – to aid fat loss – and eating so few that you no longer have the energy for running. There is no shortage of 'miracle' diets promising rapid weight loss but, in my experience, the more slowly weight comes off, the more likely it is to stay off. Rather than aiming for a specific target –1lb a week, or half a stone by the end of the month – I recommend cutting your current daily calorie intake by 15 per cent. Here's why:

Let's say you want to lose 1lb a week and continue running: 1lb of fat contains approximately 4000 calories, so to shed that weight, you need to slash 4000 calories off your weekly calorie intake – 570 calories per day. If you eat around 2000 calories per day (the recommended intake for women in the UK), that means reducing your daily intake by more than a quarter. That is very challenging, and you're likely to get tired and irritable. But let's say you decide to cut 15 per cent of your daily intake. That means reducing intake by 300 calories – a far more realistic goal and one that will enable you to continue running. It might take you a bit longer to reach your goal weight, but I can guarantee you'll get there happier, fitter and full of energy.

One final thing – don't rely on the scales for your assessment. Regular running will increase your body's lean muscle mass, and since muscle is heavier than fat, you might find that your body weight doesn't go down, or even increases. Don't worry – as long as your clothes are feeling looser, and your body fat is going down, you're winning the battle.

How to cut 15 per cent

- Downsize your portions.
- Reduce alcohol intake.
- Eat regular meals (and don't skip breakfast).
- Fill up on fibre.
- Include liquid foods, like soup and smoothies, in your diet.
- Lower your fat intake.
- Choose snacks wisely.
- Go easy on energy bars and sports drinks.

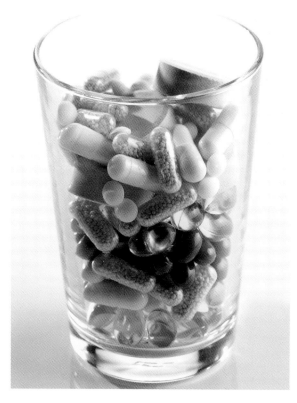

Reality check

Before you embark on a weight-loss plan, are you sure you need to lose weight? Have you checked your body mass index (BMI – see p. 23), or had your body fat measured? Although it's easy to assume that good runners should be skinny, the reality is that they come in all shapes and sizes. Most elite endurance runners have less fat than a pretzel, but this is how they were born. All of us have an optimal healthy weight and that differs from person to person. You can't force your body to be a size zero if it is naturally a size 12 any more than you can turn a pear-shaped body into an hourglass. Women have more body fat than men for a reason – to support pregnancy and lactation – and if your body fat falls below a healthy level your periods can stop, which has a detrimental effect on bone health. Women who starve themselves and train hard to get or stay skinny can end up with stress fractures, premature osteoporosis and eating disorders.

Making gains

What if you want to gain weight? The key thing is to ensure that you aren't creating a 'negative energy balance' through running, by burning off more calories than you consume. To gain weight you'll need to supply your body with more energy than it needs to maintain your current weight. Work out your TDEE (see p. 134) and then increase daily calorie intake by 15 per cent. Try to keep the percentages of your major nutrients the same, but simply increase the 'size of the pie' (the total energy expenditure).

Vitamins and minerals – a whistle-stop tour

Every woman needs an adequate intake of vitamins and minerals, and the best way to achieve this is through eating a healthy, varied and balanced diet. If you don't regularly eat at least five portions of fruit and vegetables daily, you may want to consider taking a multivitamin and mineral supplement. Bear in mind that studies suggest that deriving these micronutrients from food is better than getting them in supplements. A deficiency in a particular nutrient can harm performance, but taking more than the recommended amount won't enhance it. The evidence as to whether running women need more of certain micronutrients is mixed, but you don't want to be falling short on these, particularly iron and calcium.

Any old iron

Iron forms part of haemoglobin, which is what carries oxygen around the body, so its role is vital. Do running women need more iron? Women in general (at least, those who are premenopausal) need more than menthey lose more through menstruation. The UK guidelines are 14.8mg per day for women (8.7mg for men). It's also possible that runners need a little more than non-runners due to something called 'footstrike haemolysis', which is damage to red blood cells caused by the high impact of running (this is most likely to occur in heavier runners). More iron is also lost through the gastrointestinal tract and sweat.

We tend to think of iron deficiency as anaemia, but there is a condition called non-anaemic iron deficiency, where haemoglobin levels are normal, but ferritin (how the body stores iron) is low. This is more common in athletes, and research from the University of Missouri suggests iron supplementation can restore iron balance and improve endurance performance. That said, if you don't have an iron shortage in the first place, supplementation is unlikely to be beneficial, and excessive doses can be toxic. If you suspect you might be deficient (symptoms include fatigue, sub-par performance and 'heavy' legs) the best thing to do is to get your haemoglobin and ferritin levels tested. Vegetarians, dieters and women with heavy periods are most at risk of iron deficiencies.

To make the most of your iron intake:
- choose haem sources where possible (sources from meat and fish, rather than non-animal sources).
- avoid tea and coffee with iron-rich foods or supplements – it hampers absorption.
- eat or drink something rich in vitamin C with your iron source, to enhance absorption.

Bone up on calcium

Calcium is best known for its role in building bone and maintaining bone density as we age, but it also plays a crucial part in muscular contraction. While running is good for bone health, sweat-induced calcium loss can be higher than in non-active people. It is therefore important that you meet the intake guidelines. The UK recommended daily intake for calcium is 700mg for premenopausal women and 1000mg for breastfeeding and postmenopausal women, but guidelines in other countries are significantly higher. In the United States, postmenopausal women are recommended to take 1200mg per day, while in Australia it's 1300mg.

Good sources of calcium include all dairy products (skimmed milk is as good as full-fat), tinned bony fish like sardines and salmon, green leafy vegetables, pulses and products fortified with calcium. You'll need to look for fortified foods if you don't eat dairy, and perhaps consider supplementation.

Vitamin D also plays an important role in bone health, working closely with calcium, so ensure you get enough. Most vitamin D is derived from sunlight and it can be stored in the body, so isn't required every day, but research suggests that an increasing number of people have low levels, perhaps due to an indoor-based lifestyle. Hopefully, that means runners should be getting greater exposure, being outdoors more frequently. If you do supplement intake, avoid high doses – up to 0.025mg daily should be safe. A low intake of calcium and vitamin D has been associated with stress fractures in runners.

Go-faster foods and supplements

Myriad supplements and products claim to improve performance – from increasing fat expenditure to accelerating recovery from training and even increasing aerobic capacity. The truth is, most of them don't work. But there are a couple of exceptions. As far as endurance performance is concerned, caffeine can undoubtedly help. Studies have shown that it can improve muscular contractility (the efficiency of your muscular recruitment), reduce 'rate of perceived exertion' (RPE) and improve mental focus during prolonged activity. It can also leave you feeling jittery, irritable or with gastrointestinal distress (read about tummy troubles on p. 178). It's not necessarily for everyone (coffee addicts are unlikely to experience such a marked improvement as those who rarely drink it), but it's worth a try. Studies show that a single dose ranging from 3–6mg per kg of body weight is safe and effective – a cup of coffee typically contains 75–130mg of caffeine. Take your caffeine fix 60–75 minutes before exercise. In long events, such as the marathon, additional top-ups of a low dose (1mg per kg of body weight) can be helpful.

There's also been some exciting research on a less common beverage: beetroot juice. In 2010, researchers at the University of Exeter found that the high levels of nitrate in beetroot juice could help to reduce oxygen consumption during running, as well as improving tolerance of high-intensity exercise, increasing time to exhaustion by 15 per cent. The amount drunk in this study was 500ml per day – enough to stain your lips and dye your urine pink, but it yielded results in six days!

Tart cherry juice is another drink that is being touted for its recovery-enhancing properties. This is due to its high content of anthocyanin, a powerful antioxidant. In one study, from Northumbria University, 20 recreational marathon runners were given tart cherry juice or a placebo for five days before their race, on race day, and two days after. Those who received the cherry juice experienced less inflammation and their muscle function recovered more quickly. Other good sources of anthocyanin include blackberries, blackcurrants and blueberries.

Other plant-based compounds called polyphenols are also believed to aid recovery from hard exercise. Again, berry sources are a good bet, or try pomegranate.

Do I need more antioxidants?

While physical training increases oxidative stress in the body (which leads to the production of free radicals), it also appears to boost your body's ability to deal with it. Since antioxidants play such an important role in recovery and immune-system function, it is worth making sure you get plenty of them. Those who are most likely to be falling short are those who rely on processed foods, those who don't get their 'five a day' and those on restricted diets. The best way to maximise your intake is to eat a wide variety of fruits and vegetables – the more colourful the better. Reds, oranges and yellows are good colours to choose. The jury is still out as to whether supplementation is a good idea. If possible, stick to real food.

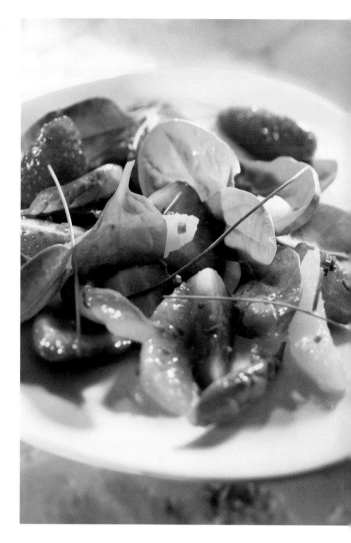

Good hydration
What and when to drink

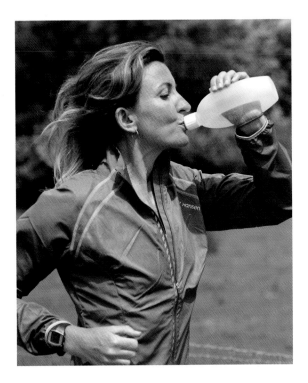

Good hydration is important whether you are sitting at your desk, negotiating the M25 or running 10km. The body doesn't operate as well when you are dehydrated, because water is at the heart of virtually every human function, from regulating body temperature to nutrient and oxygen transport, muscle contraction to joint cushioning. Plasma, which makes up 55 per cent of blood volume, is 95 per cent water; if you are dehydrated, the blood becomes thicker and the heart has to work harder to pump it around the body.

Even without exercise, we need around 1ml water for every calorie we consume (2000 calories = 2 litres water). A large proportion of our fluid needs are met by foods from cucumber and melon to bread and potatoes.

If you run regularly, though, you need more fluid to make up for the increased amount lost through sweat (the body sweats to keep body temperature constant – and that doesn't just apply to sultry days). How much more do you need? And what should that fluid be?

How much fluid is enough?

A few years ago, there were concrete guidelines regarding how much fluid to drink before, during and after a run. But in 2007, the American College of Sports Medicine (ACSM), a leading authority on exercise, revised its guidelines and no longer recommends specific volumes of fluid. This is because individual needs vary so widely that a 'one-size-fits-all' amount could result in one person drinking far too little and another drinking far too much. Typical sweat rates for a runner can range from 0.4–1.8 litres per hour. So what's a girl to do?

Start by becoming familiar with your fluid needs by monitoring your intake during training and finding out what works. There are three ways to do this – and it is best to use them all in unison:

- **Thirst** It was once claimed that when you felt thirsty, it was 'too late' to drink, meaning you were already dehydrated. But experts no longer feel there is a need to stay one step ahead of your thirst and believe it is a reliable mechanism.
- **Urine output** (both volume and colour) Are you producing a normal volume of clear or pale-coloured urine? Or is the volume scant and the shade more Tango than lemonade? If so, you may be dehydrated. University of Connecticut researchers found that urine colour correlated very accurately with hydration.

Is dehydration dangerous?

Research has shown that endurance athletes can tolerate up to 2 per cent dehydration during exercise without too many adverse effects – the water released from glycogen stores mobilised during exercise helps to account for this. That's why in the 'sweat test' (below), it is acceptable to replace only 80 per cent of what you lose, rather than 100 per cent. Higher levels of dehydration can be detrimental to your health and your running prowess. A dehydration level of 4 per cent could cause a 25 per cent drop in performance.

Pale yellow urine was indicative of being within 1 per cent of optimal hydration.

- **Common sense** When did you last have a drink? Are you running in hot sunshine? Are you sweating a lot? Applying logic to whether or not you need to drink (and how much) is perfectly valid. If your stomach is already bloated with water, don't drink more.

The sweat test

If you want to get a little more scientific about your fluid needs, the 'sweat test' gives you a snapshot of how much fluid you lose during a run – and how much to replace.

- Weigh yourself (in kilograms) naked before a training run of a measured time (30 or 60 minutes is ideal).
- Do not drink any fluid during the run.
- Towelling off excess sweat first, weigh yourself when you return (don't go to the toilet between weigh-ins).
- The amount of weight lost represents water loss – each gram equates to 1ml fluid. If you ran for 30 minutes, double the figure to get your hourly fluid loss. If you ran for 60 minutes, the figure represents your hourly fluid loss. You should aim to replace 80–100 per cent

of this fluid loss per hour during future runs, according to thirst, preference and common sense.

- Bear in mind that factors such as the temperature and your running pace will influence fluid loss. So the figure may need to be adjusted slightly up or down.

Example: before a half-hour run, you weigh 63kg. Afterwards you weigh 62.6kg. You lost 0.4kg (400g), equalling 400ml fluid. In an hour you would have lost 800ml. You would then aim to drink 640–800ml per hour when running in similar conditions.

Drinking on the run

Once you've got an idea of how much fluid you need, try breaking it down into smaller amounts. In the example above, the runner could aim to drink 160–200ml every 15 minutes during an hour-long run. (Sport scientists reckon we can absorb 175–230ml of water every 15–20 minutes). Drinking on a 'schedule' is advisable if you are one of those people who forgets to drink when you're running. Otherwise, be guided by your instinct and thirst.

Don't feel obliged to carry fluid on every run. This is only necessary when you are running for an hour or more; a shorter run isn't long enough to let the effects of dehydration take hold and affect your performance. You can simply rehydrate on your return. What is vital is avoiding starting your runs dehydrated.

What to drink

What should be in your bottle – water, fruit squash or a sports drink? The answer depends mostly on how long you are running for. Research shows quite conclusively that it is worth swapping water for an isotonic sports drink on longer runs. A Loughborough University study found that using a sports drink improved marathon times by an average of almost four minutes compared to water. But if you are trying to lose weight, bear in mind that water is calorie-free, while the average sports drink has 250 calories

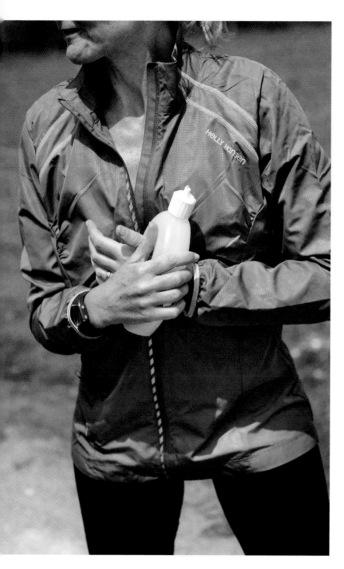

calorie-free one – contains electrolytes – salts lost in sweat, while water does not. That's helpful if you're running a long time, sweating heavily (say, in very hot conditions) or if you're a 'salty sweater' (you'll notice white 'tide marks' on your clothes).

But if you are exerting yourself on a tough run, why not use a normal sports drink, containing carbohydrates? One contention is that you'll burn more fat if you don't give your muscles a steady supply of carbohydrate. In a University of Glasgow study, 22 men cycled for one hour after an overnight fast. Half of them had a calorie-free sports drink, while the rest had a standard one. The zero-calorie group burned 41 per cent more fat. But the overall number of calories burned was the same in both groups. If you are looking to lose weight, the important factor is overall calorie expenditure, not where the calories come from. That said, those who drank the standard sports drink consumed calories while they exercised, while the calorie-free group did not. The bottom line? If you don't like water, a calorie-free sports drink is a good alternative.

But for longer runs, stick with traditional sports drinks, as the low-cal ones won't provide any fuel to your muscles.

Post-run hydration

Rehydration is one of the most important components of recovery. The body requires 3ml of water for every gram of carbohydrate it has used to restock depleted glycogen stores. The ACSM Position Stand (2007) on Hydration states that you need to drink one and a half times the amount of fluid lost during exercise to fully rehydrate afterwards. Drink little and often in the hours following your workout. Follow the guidelines on pp. 144–145 for determining what, when and how much to drink. Water is the best option, unless you have done a very long or hard run, in which case, opt for a drink that can help to fulfil all your recovery needs of carbohydrate, electrolytes, protein and fluid. There are designated 'recovery' drinks on the market, but research in 2009 concluded that chocolate milk fits the bill perfectly!

per litre. It is not necessary to consume carbohydrate during or following runs of less than 60 minutes.

The lowdown on low-calorie sports drinks

When I first heard about low-calorie sports drinks I branded them a marketing gimmick. Surely the point of a sports drink is to top up fuel levels, so if it contains virtually no carbohydrates, or is calorie-free, where's the benefit over water? The main difference is that a sports drink – even a

Sports drinks checklist

- Look for sports drinks with an 'isotonic' formula (this means it is absorbed into the bloodstream as quickly as water).
- Isotonic drinks contain 6–8 per cent carbohydrate. Any higher and a drink is no longer isotonic and would be classed as an 'energy' drink, which won't provide carbohydrate quickly enough to utilise during the run.
- A sports drink should contain electrolyte salts including sodium, potassium and chloride, which are lost through sweat.
- Choose something you like the taste of. Many of these drinks can taste overly sweet and artificial, and studies show that if you don't like the taste you won't drink enough.
- If you don't want to fork out for a branded sports drink, make your own: mix 200–250ml squash (not sugar-free) with 800ml water and add a quarter teaspoon of salt.

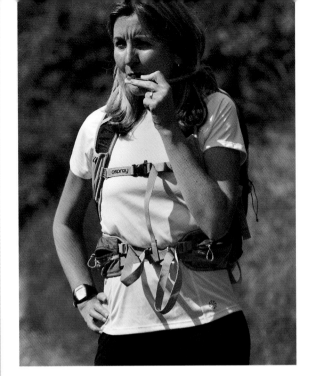

Too much of a good thing

Most runners know the importance of hydration, but it can be a matter of 'too much of a good thing'. A condition called hyponatraemia has caused a handful of fatalities and illness among runners in long-distance events like marathons and Ironman triathlons. Hyponatraemia is caused by overconsumption of water – usually drinking too much, too quickly, so that the amount drunk exceeds the amount lost through sweat. Excessive water 'dilutes' the blood, lowering its concentration of sodium – a situation exacerbated by the fact that sodium levels are also depleted through sweating. It's a double whammy – the addition of water and the removal of sodium create an abnormally, and dangerously, low level of blood sodium. Normally, if you drank excessive amounts of water, you'd wee it out. But this mechanism is less effective during exercise, with urine production declining by 20–60 per cent, lessening the opportunity of restoring sodium balance to normal. The symptoms of hyponatraemia include muscle weakness, disorientation, swollen hands and feet, headaches, nausea and breathing difficulties – in serious cases it can cause brain swelling, leading to collapse, coma and death.

It sounds alarming, but hyponatraemia is highly unlikely to be a risk for anyone who is running shorter distances and following the guidelines outlined regarding fluid intake. Those most likely to suffer hyponatraemia in long-distance events are slower runners who drink at every mile, particularly those with a smaller body size. If you are running long, and going very slow, having a salty snack can help keep sodium levels up. Using sports drinks instead of water is another smart move. But dehydration is, ultimately, a much more common problem among runners than hyponatraemia.

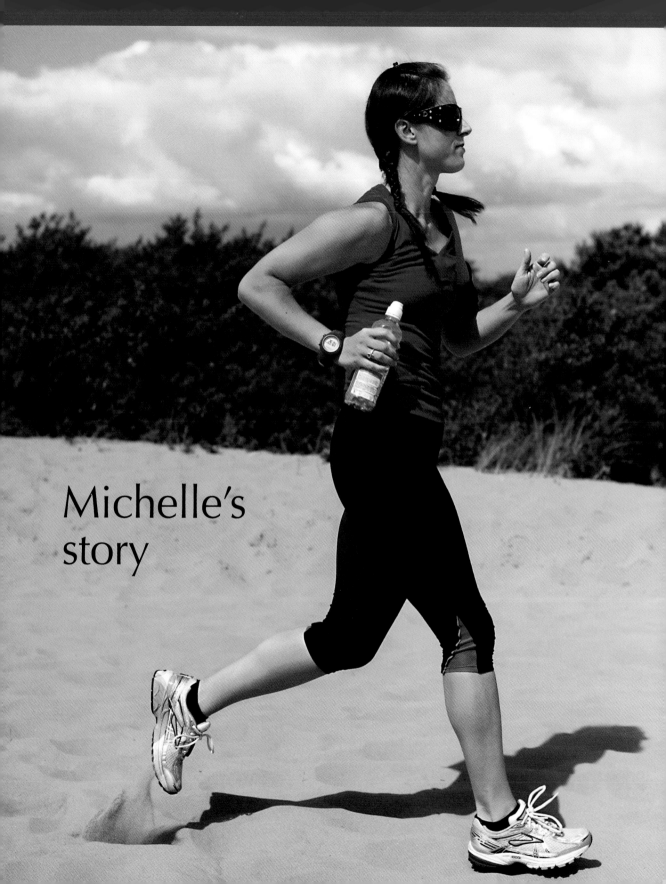

Michelle's
story

'Running has given me my life back'

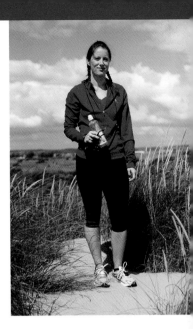

I was a fitness fanatic: in the gym four times a week doing two- to three-hour sessions, and I loved it. So when my husband and I had our first child, I didn't worry about my weight, or how I wasn't exercising any more. People always said, 'You do so much running around with kids, it will just fall off,' and I chose to believe them. Needless to say, it didn't, but I was so busy raising a child, working part-time and running a home that I didn't have time to worry about me, and how I was feeling.

When my second daughter came along in 2009, more weight piled on. I was exhausted, fat and flabby. Life became an endless routine of children, work and chores, and my confidence and self-esteem fell through the floor. Even worse, I was taking it out on my family.

The turning point came when the only size jeans I could fit into were size 18 (I am only 1.65m tall). Enough was enough! I joined a local slimming club and started doing a little exercise at home using a workout DVD; it was only half an hour, but I did it religiously three times a week and it began to work. That encouraged me to take up the longstanding offer of my best friend to go running with her. I felt so self-conscious, but it was easier having Emma by my side, and we ran a mile. I was knackered by the end of it, but I did it again, and before I knew it I was running 3–4 miles at a time, surrounded by scenic countryside. For the first time since before the children were born, I had some 'me' time.

The best thing about running is that I can do it whenever – all I need is a pair of running shoes (oh, and my husband home to look after the kids). I still have a house to run, a job to do and two children to raise, but running has given me my life back. Everyone has commented on what a different person I am. It has helped me to lose the extra weight (I am now 23kg lighter) but, more importantly, I've regained what I lost – my self-esteem, my confidence, my body!

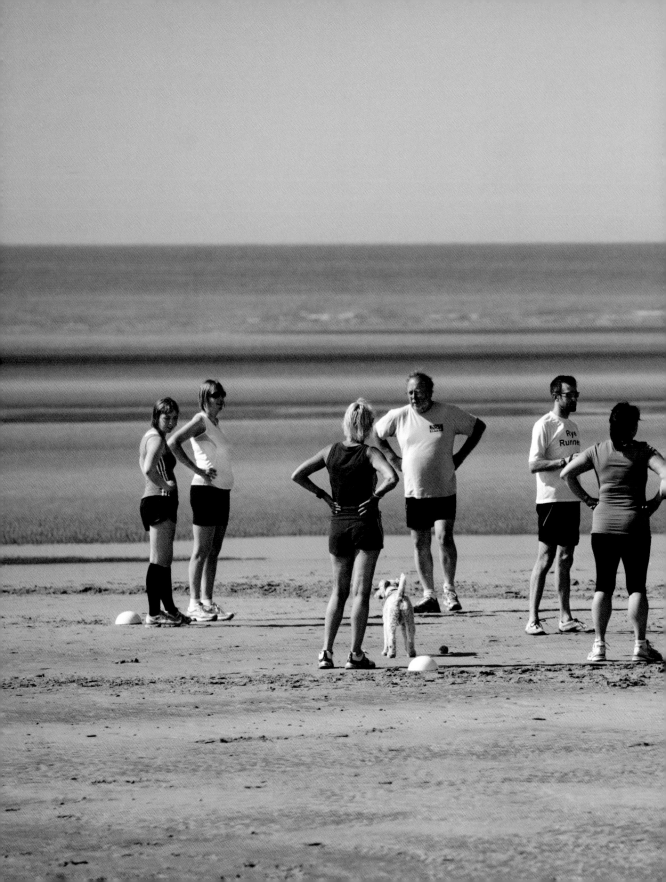

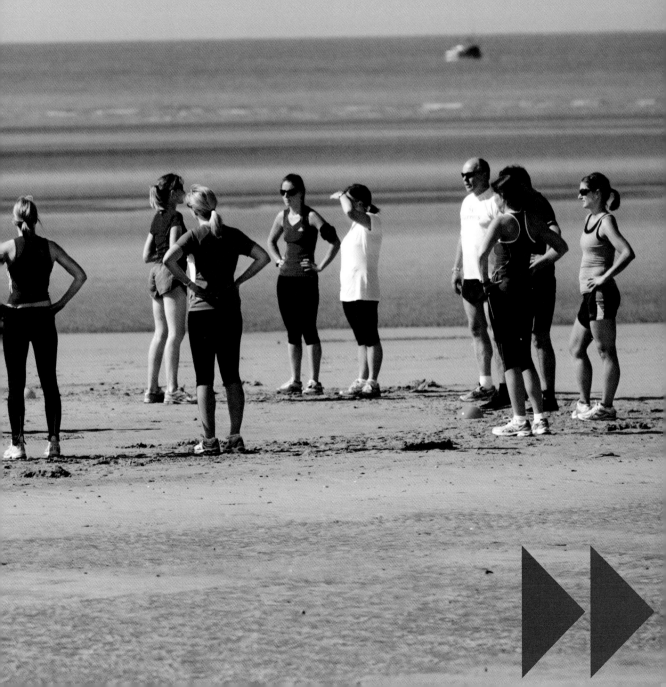

The human race

Running together
Joining the running community

I love to run alone, but I also love the camaraderie of running with others: the chance to catch up with a good friend, the witty banter on my Saturday morning group runs, the team spirit on a training holiday...

Sharing your running (with the right people) makes it more fun, introduces an element of competition and offers support and encouragement. A 2009 Oxford University study found that exercising with others produces more endorphins than exercising alone, elevating mood and promoting a sense of social bonding. It doesn't have to involve physically running with someone else – the burgeoning number of online 'communities' enables you to be part of something, even if you run alone.

Clubs and groups

There are running clubs to be found almost everywhere – from big cities to rural villages. Most are affiliated to UK Athletics, the governing body for running in the UK, but if there isn't an 'official' athletics club, there may be a club operating from your local gym or running shop or a group of like-minded people who train together.

I'd like to tell you that running clubs welcome everyone – regardless of ability, age, shape or size – but unfortunately, this is not always true. Recently, a woman I coached who has moved to a different area told me that she telephoned her local running club to enquire about joining and was asked how old she was and how much she weighed. As if to justify his questions, the man explained, 'The thing is, we have some women who turn up and weigh 14 stone – ridiculous!' Another lady I know, who was progressing so well in my weekly sessions that she'd decided to get an additional run in with the local club was abandoned on the streets of London in the evening

because the regulars didn't bother to wait for her. And clubs wonder why new members don't come – or stay. But there are many great clubs out there who do offer beginners support, encouragement and a friendly welcome. So if you don't find it at the first place you try, keep looking.

There are a couple of other options worth checking out. Women on the Run is a female-only organisation with groups operating across England. Their ethos is to be all-inclusive, and the emphasis is very much on getting started in a fun, supportive and safe environment – although many members do go on to compete in races. Research from the Medical College of Georgia in Augusta found that same-sex environments helped women who were self-conscious about exercise to stick with it and enjoy it more. In a similar vein – but not exclusively for women – is UK Athletics' Run England. This was set up to offer beginners intimidated by the club system a chance to get started. Before you join any running group, speak to someone there, check out their website or pay a visit to get a feel for how friendly it is, whether there are runners at your level, how competitive it is (some clubs like their members to race regularly) and what – if any – kind of expertise is available in the way of coaching and training programmes. For UK Athletics clubs, you pay an annual fee to join, but this entitles you to enter races at a reduced rate and you generally won't pay for sessions on top. Many other groups charge a small weekly fee, although some are free. See Resources, p. 205 for more information.

Running online

Don't relish the presence of other runners? Online running communities enable you to get advice, swap tips and

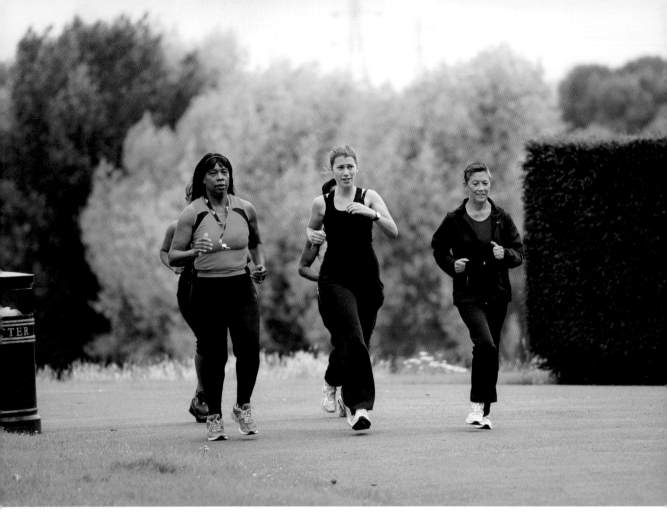

Seven reasons to join a club

1   It's a great way of finding new routes.
2   Meet new training partners.
3   Get access to expert coaching.
4   Unearth your competitive streak!
5   It's safer running with others.
6   Running at a fixed time makes you more likely to stick to it.
7   It's easier to do speed work when someone else is timing you.

share support with runners around the globe when it suits you. This can be useful; a runner might post a question like, 'I'm thinking of doing the Bath Half Marathon – is it beginner-friendly?' and get some insightful responses. As with any social networking, you're going to have to trawl through a lot of chatter to find the good stuff. *Runner's World* magazine operates one of the most useful and active online forums, where 'threads' (an ongoing conversation about a specific topic) include beginners, injuries and clubs; there's even a 'pregnant runners club'. The site is the best race resource in the UK, with detailed information and reader ratings. Another good resource is Fetcheveryone, a free website for runners (with a growing number of triathletes, cyclists and swimmers). You can use it simply as an online training log but it is a very social site, with member banter, forum discussion and a real 'club' feel. You can start your own blog about your training on the site or get advice and inspiration from other members and via the weekly newsletter and articles. There is a useful race finder, and you can log race results; there's a weekly 'league table', showing members' fastest times, PBs and age-related rankings. You have to sign up though – it's strictly members only.

There are also thousands of running blogs and websites online. The quality varies enormously, as does the subject matter, so target your search to whatever it is you are specifically looking for, be it ultra running, injury or stretching. I recommend a degree of caution when you're researching a topic online – don't take everything you read as gospel, especially regarding injury. The people giving the advice may be no more experienced than you are.

Running holidays and camps

Given that I met my husband on a training camp, I couldn't neglect to mention the advantages of running holidays! The beauty of a training camp is that you have nothing to worry about except for eating, sleeping and training, giving you a great opportunity to focus on your running. If you've picked well, you'll gain invaluable feedback and advice from qualified coaches. Many people go alone, so don't worry if you don't have a like-minded friend or partner. Before you book, make sure that you have a good idea of the standard of running expected, including the volume of training planned and the terrain. Will participants be divided into different ability groups? Is there any actual coaching/feedback on your technique? Some camps have specific themes – most popularly, marathon training. Others combine running with other activities, like yoga. If your training camp is also your holiday, check out the standard of the facilities and the food and accommodation options (these range from 'no frills' to deluxe). Find out what there is to do in the area if you plan to take a day off.

The world's biggest running club

NikePlus claims to be the 'largest running club in the world' with more than 4 million members. To be a part of it, you need to have a NikePlus sports kit, which consists of a sensor which fits inside your shoe (or to the shoelaces) and a receiver, which plugs into your iPod, iPod Touch, iPhone or a Nike SportBand. After your run, you plug the receiver into a computer to download your running data to your 'home page' on the site. This is the gateway to the millions of other members, with whom you can chat, compare performances, set or take part in challenges. You can set yourself goals (there are pre-set programmes for specific distances or you can tailor-make your own programme) and track your progress.

Once you are actually 'on camp', it's easy to get sucked into doing a lot more training than normal. It's partly because you have more time available, but peer pressure is also a factor. Establish your boundaries before you go, so you don't risk coming home exhausted or harbouring an injury. A good way to dip your toes in the water is by going on a training weekend, to get a feel for whether a longer camp is for you. See Resources, p. 205 for recommended training camp operators.

Getting a coach

A few years ago, getting a running coach was only for those planning to compete at a high level – but nowadays, it is recognised that coaching can be beneficial for all runners. There are a few options. Many coaches offer a tailor-made programme online, by email, post or phone,

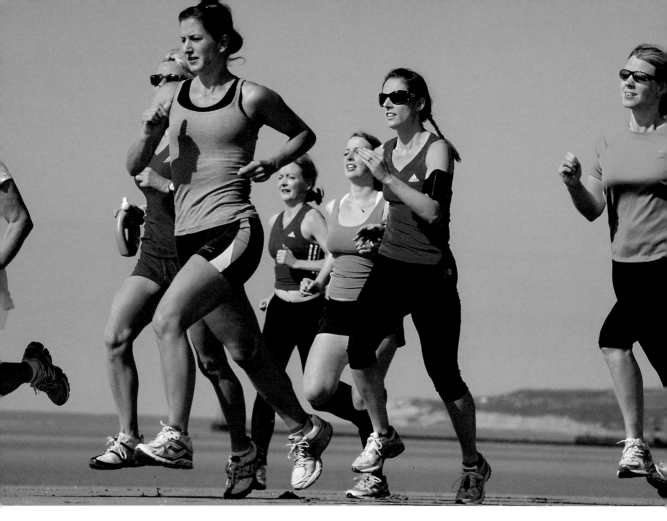

which is based on the information you give them about your running status and your goals. This can work really well when you are training for a specific event. Other coaches offer one-to-one sessions, which are particularly useful if you want to improve your technique or need guidance on how to tackle speed or hill sessions. Group workshops are another option – these tend to focus on technique or race preparation. There is no central resource where you can search for a coach, so contact your local running club, look online or ask other runners for recommendations. Make sure you pick someone who is suitably qualified and experienced, but also someone who you get on with and who understands your needs.

> "
>
> Joining a running club might appear daunting, but it's worth it. I've made great friends through our small running club. We email daily, run together, congratulate and commiserate over achievements or injuries, encourage and spur each other on.
>
> Fiona

Four-legged training partners

A dog can make the perfect running partner – providing company, security and added fun. But not all dogs make good distance runners. It's down to the breed, but also the individual dog's preferences and previous experience. My fox terrier, Sidney, is one of my favourite and longest-standing running partners. At ten years old, he's not as speedy as he once was, nor does he have the staying power for long runs, but he still enjoys shorter outings. Sometimes I have to cajole, encourage and flatter him every step of the way, other times he bounds ahead like a puppy – but since there's no predicting how he'll feel, I take him only on runs where it won't matter if I stop and start, or even walk for a bit, so that I don't get frustrated or push him too hard. I also stick to softer surfaces to protect his joints. Sid runs best off-lead, but I find a waist-mounted lead with bungee cord invaluable for when he needs one (see Resources, p. 205).

If you are thinking of taking your dog for a run, start with a very short session to see how he fares. He, too, needs to build his 'training' up gradually. He can't inform you if he's struggling; dogs want to please you, so be watchful of signs of over-exertion, such as excessive panting, a dry tongue or simply slowing down. Avoid running on hot days – dogs can't regulate their body temperature on the move as efficiently as humans. And remember to carry some water with you or run via a place where he can take a drink. Dogs under six months shouldn't go on sustained runs; wait until their bones and muscles are fully developed. If your dog is overweight or mature, check with your vet before taking him running.

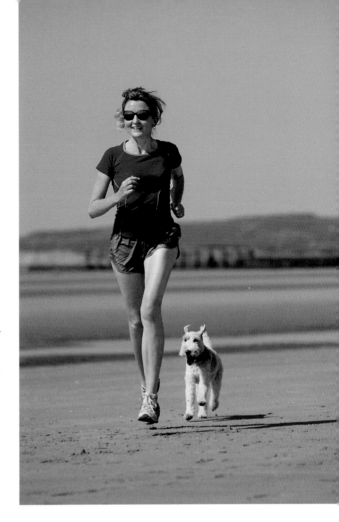

I started running when I got my first dog, Rufus. He needed a great deal of exercise and I soon realised I could fit an exercise routine into my week more easily if I turned dog walking into running.

Helen B

Staying power
Running through thick and thin

If I were to tell you that I am filled with excitement every time I lace up my trainers, and return from every run glowing with energy, I would be lying. Motivation ebbs and flows, and the secret – most of the time – is getting yourself to go, even when you don't feel like it. I say most of the time because there are occasions when it's better to give running a miss. So how can you persuade yourself to don trainers instead of slippers?

Just do it

It has become a well-worn axiom, but research suggests you are better off just getting on with your workout, rather than thinking about it. In a 2011 study, published in the journal *Health Psychology*, more than 200 people interviewed prior to and after a workout greatly underestimated how much they would enjoy exercising. The researchers dub this 'forecasting myopia' – the notion that when we contemplate exercise we recall only the first few minutes, which tend to be the toughest. If we can recall and focus on how good we feel during (or after) a run, we maximise our likelihood of making it a reality.

Ask 'What if?'

When you're struggling with motivation, ask yourself: 'What will happen if I don't go?' and 'What will happen if I do go?' The chances are, you'll feel annoyed and disappointed if you don't go.

Put your kit on

Devastatingly simple, but effective! A runner gave me this tip years ago and I've used it with repeated success. At

> When I hit the wall on a run, I begin to count backwards from a number equal to the number of metres remaining. On a 5km run last year, I reached 4km and banished thoughts of stopping by counting 1000, 999, 998... I soon realised, metres from the finish line, that I had both lost count and forgotten any sense of defeat!
>
> Mary

the very least, I'll do some strength training or stretching before taking my running clothes off, but generally it gets me out running.

Make a small commitment

Running programmes provide structure and focus. But they aren't the be-all and end-all. If you can't face what's set out in the schedule, what can you handle? Ten minutes? Twenty minutes? Pledge to do just a little running and if you don't feel like carrying on after that, then you can go home feeling good that you tried instead of staying home feeling guilty.

Imagine

When you are debating whether to go for a run, visualise yourself approaching the front door at the end of a great session, feeling re-energised. Or create a vivid mental image of yourself out on one of your favourite routes – picture the scenery, feel the rhythm of your feet, smell the spring flowers. Then see if you're not tempted! You can also use visualisation to keep yourself focused during a race: picture the finish and you running towards it, feeling fast and strong.

Dear diary

I started writing down what I'd done the first week I went running, over 20 years ago. Every year since, I've kept a record of the sessions I've done (including other exercise) and recorded anything I think might be important, such as any niggles or if I was very tired or felt particularly good. I mention if I've tried a new pair of shoes or brand of sports drink. I'll write my distance and time and, if it was a high-intensity session, what my pace was during the efforts.

There are three main benefits to keeping a diary. Firstly, it makes you feel accountable. It's as if your training journal is waiting for you to fill it with all your sessions,

> "
> When I don't feel like going out for a run (which is quite a lot of the time), I find it's useful to have organised to go with someone else a few days in advance, so I'm committed – then I can't back out as easily. I enjoy it when I get going!
> Clare
> "

and you feel a bit guilty if you don't have anything to report! Secondly, it provides information to help shape your training. You might notice that you didn't do many long runs in the lead-up to a disappointing 10km race, and schedule in more for next time. Or you might see that the niggle in your Achilles tendon began when you started going to the track to do speed work. These 'clues' can be really helpful in monitoring what works for you. Thirdly, your diary can really be useful as a powerful motivator. You can look back and see that in January you could hardly make it to the park without walking. Now you run there, do two laps and run back. What progress!

There are lots of high-tech options for keeping a training journal, from online logs that your HRM or GPS watch can download data to wirelessly, to smart phone apps and websites. There are also designated training journals available, with space for various details, from your daily heart rate and weight to the weather. Use whatever works for you.

When not to run

Everyone has down days, and often we can push through them. But if you've experienced a consistent dip in your fitness that can't be explained by illness or injury, and you dread training sessions that you used to enjoy, it's likely that you are suffering from burnout or 'over-training'. It might sound like something that only affects elite athletes on a twice-a-day, seven-days-a-week schedule, but it isn't. It's possible for you to be pushing as hard as an elite athlete, relative to your own genetic limitations. Athletes are innately gifted, but they also schedule 'down time'. They rest, eat properly and train correctly – and, even then, most don't get through the year injury-free. They also have the expertise of coaches, physiotherapists and nutritionists to support them.

Don't beat yourself up, thinking: 'I could cope before; why not now?' You may have been laying the foundations of over-training for some time. Your training capacity isn't set in concrete. Five training sessions a week might be fine

How to keep going...when the going gets tough

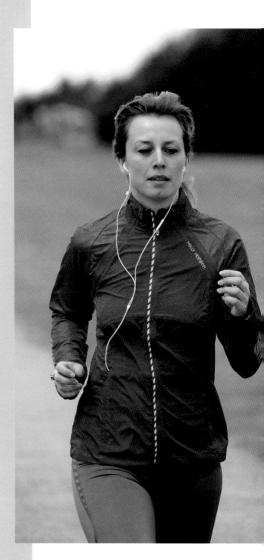

Getting out the door can sometimes be an achievement in itself – but how do you keep going when fatigue or discomfort are telling you to give up?

- **Listen to music** The research on the effects of music on performance is compelling. Studies have shown music can distract you from fatigue, prolong endurance and enhance motor skills. The best choice is music that enables you to synchronise your work rate to the tempo – a beat with the same rhythm as your footstrike. You have to like the music for it to work, though, so create a playlist of songs that inspire you. That said, I never listen to music when I run; I much prefer to tune into my surroundings. Sometimes I use music before I run to rev myself up.

- **Tune in, zone out** Sport psychologists identify two different types of 'attentional strategy' – association and dissociation. Association means turning your attention inwards, focusing on your body – the rhythm of your breathing, the sound of your feet landing; dissociation is the opposite – turning your attention outwards on to external distractions, like music, planning a presentation at work or looking in shop windows. While everyone has their own preferred strategy, both types can be useful at different times. A study in the journal *Sports Medicine* found that dissociative strategies were more effective in reducing perception of effort and enhancing mood at low- to moderate-exercise intensities. But their effectiveness isn't so great during high-intensity effort, when physiological cues – like your heart pounding – usually dominate. It's also been suggested that associative strategies help you to regulate intensity, helping to avoid injury or overexertion. In a study from the University of Otago in New Zealand, runners were told their heart rate and oxygen uptake as they ran on a treadmill. Then they were taught relaxation techniques to use while running. After six weeks of practice, the runners were able to lower their heart rate and oxygen uptake at the same pace by implementing the relaxation techniques.

- **Have a mantra** A mantra is a word or short phrase used to keep your mind trained on what you're doing, rather than thinking 'this hurts' or 'I'm too tired to carry on'. It can work wonders if your mind is feeding you negative thoughts while you're running. A couple of examples: 'strong and steady' and 'I am running fast and strong'. A mantra should consist of positive words and focus on something within your control.

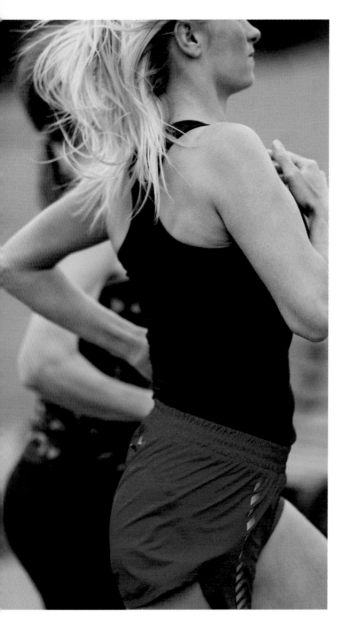

most of the time, but it can become too much if the kids are on holidays, if work is stressful or if you're sleeping badly. If you're feeling burned out, back off. At the very least, reduce your training volume, but, if necessary, take a week or two off altogether. You'll almost certainly come back stronger.

Falling off the wagon – and getting back on

There are a couple of women in my running group who I'd assumed were beginners. It turned out that one had run a marathon a few years before, the other had run a half marathon. Another woman came religiously for a few weeks, achieved a 10km and then disappeared. So what makes us give up?

Sometimes life gets in the way – and if that's the case, the advice in this book on planning and organising should help, as will having clearly defined goals. But sometimes, it's down to our beliefs about ourselves. You can't leave your brain out of the equation when trying to change your body. If you see yourself as an 'unfit' or 'overweight' person, you may subconsciously believe that running isn't what someone like you 'does', so you don't keep it up. If you've tried before to get more active, and not succeeded, you may embark on your next attempt with the belief that it probably won't work. The chances are, with this mindset, it won't.

What's to be done? Perhaps, you think, 'I just need to be stronger' or 'I need to force myself to stick with it.' That might work for a while, but I think there's a subtle difference between willpower and motivation. Willpower is the ability to control your behaviour, but motivation is the desire to do so. Without that desire to run, it will be much harder to maintain your regime. You need to look at what you'll gain from running to find reasons to want to do it. Sport psychologists call this 'intrinsic motivation' because rather than feeling pressured or obliged to achieve something, your motivation comes from within. The best type of motivation isn't fixed on the outcome, but the process itself. Research shows that process-oriented people are better stickers than those who only focus on the result.

If you can barely remember when your last run was, trying to pin down what caused you to give up will help you get back on track. Write down what made you stop running. Was it an injury or a niggling pain that wouldn't go away? Were you constantly exhausted and lacking in energy for the next run? Had you achieved a goal and not set a new one? Be really specific when you write down what made you stop.

For each reason try to find a way of preventing that 'block' from happening again. You might jot down 'I ended up aching all over'. Possible solutions? 'I'll start a bit more cautiously next time and progress more slowly. I could run on the grass instead of the pavements.'

If your barrier to running is injury, read about injury prevention and dealing with injuries on p. 110 and p. 174. Do you need to rethink your footwear? Are you making time for strength and flexibility work? Did you allow enough time to recover from the injury before you started running again? Address these issues and you'll stop repeating the same mistakes.

Next, think about what you enjoyed about running and why you are considering – or trying – to get back into it. Did you love the inner glow it gave you? Did you like eating what you liked without gaining weight? Did you relish escaping from hassles on a Sunday morning? Try to conjure up vivid images of yourself enjoying a run and how it felt. It's a matter of finding the way back to that point from where you are now. Here are some tips that may help:

- Imagine building a wall. You put one brick down and it falls off and cracks. What do you do? Knock the entire wall down or pick up another brick and continue building? It's the same with your running. A setback – whether it's a week or a month – doesn't signal the end of everything. Get back on track when you can and don't try to make up for lost time by

> "
> I used to go to my weekly Parkrun thinking, 'I'm going to try to beat my time'. If I succeeded, I got a great sense of achievement afterwards, but it meant putting a lot of pressure on myself. One time, I decided to change my thought to 'I love to run fast'. I looked at the trees, felt the wind in my hair, smiled and thoroughly enjoyed the run. At the end, I'd knocked a minute off my PB.
>
> Sarah H
> "

launching into a punishing schedule.

- Leave your watch at home. Concentrate on the pleasure of running without worrying about time, pace or distance. Simply run. I found this really hard when I returned to running after a long injury-related break. I kept looking at my GPS and gasping, 'How slow?' Running without it for a few weeks, letting my body dictate the pace, was the solution.
- Do not allow yourself to be pressured by others, whether it's a training partner, a running club or a coach. Only you know when you feel ready to run.
- See running as a choice, not a duty. If it feels like a chore, you need to rethink your training. Although you should feel committed to running, it should never end up being another stress in your life.
- Even if you run once or twice a week it's still once or twice more than most people. Don't beat yourself up over the runs you are missing, but congratulate yourself on those you are completing.

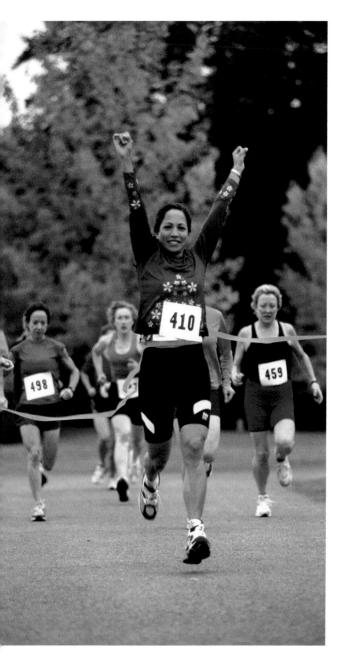

Taking part in a race may be the farthest thing from your mind when you start running, but you'd be surprised how many women, initially adamant that they aren't interested in competing, find themselves in a race – often sooner, rather than later. It might be the drip-drip feed of other runners discussing their weekend races, it might be wanting to help a charity or it may simply be that the time has come to test yourself.

Whatever your motivation, don't be put off by the notion that races are only for those who want to win – most runners are competing primarily against themselves, aiming to better their previous performances or monitor their progress.

The ideal distance to consider for your debut is 5km or 10km. Even if you have your sights set on a half or full marathon make sure you've tackled these distances first to gain valuable race experience and determine whether your long-term goal needs to be adjusted or postponed.

First race fears

Choose your first race carefully. You want it to be memorable for the right reasons. While fears about coming last are generally unfounded, if you're worried that you'll be miles off the back, contact the organisers for an honest opinion. In general, races organised by running clubs will be faster than those arranged by commercial companies. Some races have a cut-off time, which indicates the slowest expected finish times. You can also look up previous years' results to see the slowest and fastest times and get a feel for whether this is a race you'll be comfortable in. If you like the idea of a female-only event, the options are growing. The nationwide Race for Life series continues to burgeon and offers the ideal opportunity to lose your race virginity – it's fun, friendly and supportive and you should be able to find one close to home. Here are some other important factors to consider:

- **Don't go it alone** Sign up with a friend or training partner; you don't have to run together, but it's nice to have someone to share the pre-race nerves with…

- **What is the terrain like?** Find out if the route is off-road or on tarmac. Is it flat or hilly?

- **How many people** (the size of the 'field')? Bigger is generally better for your first race, as large events usually have plenty of first-timers. However, a bigger field makes it harder to fight your way through, should you want to.

- **Time and place** What time does the race start? Will you have a long journey to get there? If so, is that feasible with the start time? Also consider the time of year. Are you accustomed to running in summer heat or icy wind?

- **Chip timing** Many Races have 'chip timing', whereby an electronic chip, worn around your ankle or attached to your shoelaces, records your start and finish time; if you get delayed at the start your time will still be accurate. This is probably more important for subsequent races, when you might want to beat your PB.

- **The reward** There's nothing like having a medal placed around your neck! Most races give finishers medals, though some now offer alternatives like a T-shirt or other memento. Find out what's in store, if it's important to you.

Finding out about races

You can find out about races online and in running magazines like *Runner's World*, which has listings of events a few months ahead (see Resources, p. 205). The organiser's description is useful, but so are online forums, where runners 'rate' and review races. Keep an eye on gym or sports club noticeboards and your local paper too.

Once you've chosen your race, enter in advance. This increases your chances of getting a place and avoids the stress of registering on the day; better to turn up with your race number in your bag and entrance fee paid. Entering in advance also increases your commitment level, and enables you to prepare specifically for the distance to maximise your chances of a great performance.

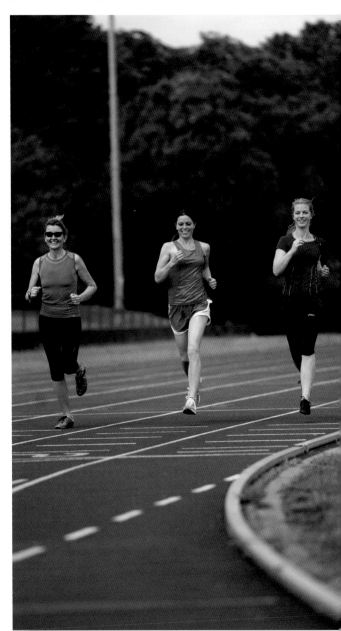

Your first race

The programmes in this section are designed to prepare you for your first 5 or 10km race. They follow the principles outlined in Chapter 4, and both programmes assume you are running regularly. I've allowed six weeks for a 5km and eight for a 10km.

How to follow the programmes

- If you don't want to train five days per week, skip the Monday run. If two high-intensity sessions per week feels too much, alternate between the Tuesday and Thursday runs.

- For the interval training sessions on Tuesdays and Thursdays, begin with at least ten minutes of easy running before you start and finish with ten minutes of easy running to cool down.

- Short intervals (Tuesdays): aim for RPE level 4 or 90–99 per cent of your maximum heart rate (see p. 68). Walk or jog the recoveries. Stick to the lower end of the suggested number of repetitions if you are new to interval training.

- Long intervals (Thursdays): aim for RPE level 3 or 82–90 per cent of your maximum heart rate. It should feel 'comfortably hard'. Walk or jog the recoveries.

- Cross-train means do an alternative activity. Try something that doesn't put too much impact on your joints, such as swimming, cycling, weight-training, yoga or Pilates. Or try the strength and stability workouts in Chapter 5.

- 'Race pace' means the pace you would like to run on the big day. Predict your 5km race pace by adding 15–40 seconds to your 1 mile (1.6km) time trial result. If, for example, you complete your mile in 8.45 your 5km race pace would be 9–9.40 per mile. You can experiment with this in training to get a feel for the right pace.

- Predict your 10km race pace from the 5km time trial by multiplying your time by two and adding one to two minutes.

Gearing up for race day

As the race draws nearer, there are a few things you can do to ensure you are well prepared. In the final few days, wind your training down. A few days is fine for a race of this length, but you would need seven to ten days to wind down for a half marathon and 14–21 days for a full one. This pre-race period is called the 'taper' and its purpose is to ensure that you reach the start line feeling fit and fresh, not exhausted. Don't be tempted to cram in extra training sessions: they will only make you more tired rather than contributing to your fitness.

Try to get plenty of rest in the week preceding the race, and it won't matter too much if you have a sleepless night the day before. Stay hydrated by drinking little and often, so that you don't toe the line dehydrated. There is no need to increase your carbohydrate intake in preparation for a 5km or 10km – your body will have enough stored, and given that you'll be training less in the last few days, you should be well stocked already. Do make sure you are getting a healthy, balanced diet – see Chapter 7. Don't skip breakfast on race morning – the body uses up around 300 calories during sleep, so top up energy with a light breakfast. Opt for something tried and tested.

Plan your route to the race. If you are driving, where are you going to park? If you are going by public transport, have you checked it's running normally? Plan a contingency option, in case something goes wrong.

Familiarise yourself with the route. If you know where the hills or tight bends are, you'll be more prepared for them. You can also figure out where to tell your 'fans' to stand to cheer you on!

Make a list of everything you'll need on race day – from your running shoes to your race number and safety pins, a drink, sunglasses (or waterproof!). When you're packing, tick everything off, so you don't forget anything.

Make firm plans with your friends and family to meet at the end. 'I'll see you at the finish' isn't a good idea in big events, as there could be hundreds of other runners. Arrange a specific place and time to meet.

5KM TRAINING PROGRAMME

WEEK	1	2	3	4	5	6
MONDAY	Easy run 20–30 mins	Easy run 30 mins	Easy run 30 mins	Easy run 30–40 mins	Easy run 30–40 mins	Easy run 20–30 mins
TUESDAY	Short intervals: 8–10 x 1 min fast, 1 min slow	Short intervals: 8–10 x 1 min fast, 1 min slow	6–10 x 2 mins fast, 2 mins slow	6–10 x 2 mins fast, 2 mins slow	4–8 x 3 mins fast, 2 mins slow	6 x 1 min fast, 1 min slow
WEDNESDAY	Rest	Rest	Rest	Rest	Rest	Rest
THURSDAY	10 mins easy then 3 x 5 mins at threshold pace with 1 min jog/walk in between. 10 mins easy	10 mins easy then 3 x 6 mins at threshold pace with 1 min jog/walk in between. 10 mins easy	10 mins easy then 2 x 8 mins at threshold pace with 2 mins jog/walk in between. 10 mins easy	10 mins easy then 2 x 8 mins at threshold pace with 2 mins jog/walk in between. 10 mins easy	10 mins easy then 12–15 mins at race pace. 10 mins easy	Steady run 30 mins – last 5 mins at race pace.
FRIDAY	Easy run 30 mins	Steady run 30 mins	Easy run 40 mins	Steady run 40 mins	Rest	15–20-min jog
SATURDAY	Rest or cross-train	Rest or cross-train	Rest or cross-train	Rest or cross-train	Rest or cross-train	Rest
SUNDAY	Longer run 45 mins: try to run the 2nd half slightly faster than the first.	Longer run 50 mins: try to run the 2nd half slightly faster than the first.	Long run 60 mins	15 mins easy then 1 mile time trial.	Long run 60 mins: try to run the 2nd half slightly faster than the first.	RACE DAY!

10KM TRAINING PROGRAMME

WEEK	1	2	3	4	5	6	7	8
MONDAY	Easy run 30 mins	Easy run 30 mins	Easy run 30 mins	Easy run 30–40 mins	Easy run 30–40 mins	Easy run 30–40 mins	Easy run 30–40 mins	Easy run 20 mins or rest
TUESDAY	6–10 x 2 mins fast, 2 mins slow	Short intervals: 6–10 x 2 mins fast, 2 mins slow	Short intervals: 4–8 x 3 mins fast, 2 mins slow	Short intervals: 4–8 x 3 mins fast, 2 mins slow	Short intervals: 3–5 x 4 mins fast, 3 mins slow	Short intervals: 3–5 x 4 mins fast, 3 mins slow	6–10 x 1 min fast, 1 min slow	10 mins easy then 25 mins at threshold pace. 10 mins easy
WEDNESDAY	Rest	Rest	Rest	Rest	Rest	Rest	Rest	Rest
THURSDAY	10 mins easy then 4 x 5 mins at threshold pace with 1 min jog/walk in between. 10 mins easy	10 mins easy then 15 mins at threshold pace. 10 mins easy	10 mins easy then 4 x 6 mins at threshold pace with 1 min jog/walk in between. 10 mins easy	10 mins easy then 20 mins at threshold pace. 10 mins easy	10 mins easy then 4 x 8 mins at threshold pace with 90 secs jog/walk in between. 10 mins easy	10 mins easy then 25 mins at threshold pace. 10 mins easy	10 mins easy then 3 x 10 mins at threshold pace with 2 mins in between. 10 mins easy	Steady run 30 mins – last 5 mins at race pace.
FRIDAY	Easy run 40 mins	Steady run 40 mins	Easy run 45 mins	Steady run 45 mins	Easy run 30 mins	Steady run 45 mins	Easy run 45 mins	Rest
SATURDAY	Rest or cross-train	Rest or cross-train	Rest or cross-train	Rest	Rest or cross-train	Rest or cross-train	Rest or cross-train	15–20-min jog or rest
SUNDAY	Longer run 50 mins easy	Longer run 60 mins easy	Longer run 60 mins: try to run 2nd half slightly faster than the first.	5km time trial or race.	Long run 70 mins – last 5 mins at race pace.	Long run 70 mins	Long run 60 mins: try to run the 2nd half slightly faster than the first.	RACE DAY!

Parkrun

If you are still daunted by the idea of a race, but would like to test yourself over a set distance, check out Parkrun. Parkrun offers a UK-wide series of weekly 5km events and is fun, friendly and free! Although there are some serious athletes at the front in many events, parkruns aren't races – it's just you against the clock. 'The focus is on participation,' says creator Paul Sinton-Hewitt. 'We invite everyone from children to grannies to take part, and pride ourselves on the supportive, community feel of the events.' Dogs and buggies are also welcomed. Once you've signed up (register online for free), you get a personal barcode which you can use at any Parkrun – there are more than 50 locations to choose from and the network is still growing. To find out if there's a Parkrun in your area visit www.parkrun.com.

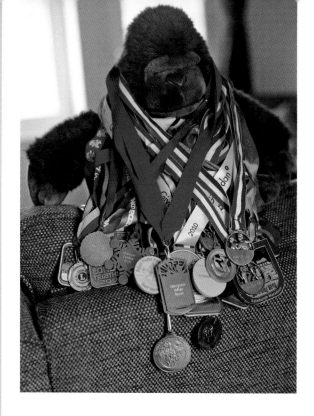

As an older runner (I am in my late 60s) who has never run more than a few miles at a time, I have no desire to start running marathons, but this doesn't mean I can't try something new. I recently discovered Parkrun. I find the distance of 5km quite manageable and am now working on trying to improve my PB.

Elly

Winning the mental game

It's perfectly normal to have butterflies, but you want them to be flying in formation! To keep nerves under control, focus on what you've achieved in training and commit to enjoying the race, regardless of your time.

If you prefer to have some time alone prior to a race, don't be persuaded to allow your family to come and stand with you. It'll only interrupt your concentration. Equally, if you are a bag of nerves and want some moral support, make sure you've got a friend or fellow runner to go with.

There's a lot of research to suggest that mental state prior to a race affects performance, so it's essential to have the right mindset. One way of getting in the zone is to create a 'pre-performance ritual'. It sounds very exotic, but it simply means devising a routine that you practise in training and always do before a race. Once the pre-performance ritual is complete, it acts as a mental 'trigger' which tells you: 'Time to go.' Or try visualisation: use all your senses to create a vivid image of yourself crossing the finish with a big smile on your face.

> Stick to what you know – race day isn't the time to start experimenting with new sports drinks, kit or wearing a running water-pack if you haven't done it in training.
>
> Emma

some plastic cups on a table in the garden. The trick is to shut your epiglottis (the 'flap' which closes the entrance to the windpipe) while you take water in your mouth, then swallow.

- If you're flagging, focus on your technique and posture. Keep your head up and your feet turning over quickly. Don't think about the finish, and how far away it is, just concentrate on taking the next step and the next one…A mantra can help focus the mind or distract you from fatigue and discomfort (see p. 159).
- When you cross the finish, don't stop suddenly. Keep moving while your heart rate and breathing rate return to normal. Don't forget to stretch (unless your muscles are very sore and tender, in which case it's best to leave stretching for another day).
- Refuel as soon as possible. You'll have been working at a hard pace in a race, so will have used a considerable amount of carbohydrate, which you should replace, along with some fluid and antioxidants. It's a good idea to take a post-race snack with you, rather than waiting till you get home or relying on what's on offer at the race.

Race day success

Here are my top tips for a successful race:

- Don't get there too early. You don't want to rush or be late, but many people over-compensate and end up standing around getting nervous and cold, when they could have had an extra half hour in bed.
- Allow time to warm up – you don't want to waste racing minutes on your warm-up pace. Jog until your heart rate reaches a steady rate and your body feels warm, and do some mobility exercises. If you have time, include some strides (see p. 44).
- Do not start off faster than your planned pace. In the excitement of the moment, it's very easy to race off, only to end up with a stitch or legs like jelly. It's dispiriting to slow down or get overtaken. Stick to your planned pace and the chances are you'll be doing the overtaking.
- Don't stop to drink. You'll need to practise this in training. You can lose valuable seconds stopping to pick up a drink and drinking it; but if you haven't got the hang of swallowing on the move, you could end up having a coughing fit, which will lose even more time. Practise drinking on the move by laying out

> I dedicate different miles to certain people, so I don't let them down by stopping or slowing up. It's all about little confidence tricks you can draw on when the going gets tough.
>
> Joan

Marathon woman

You don't have to be under 35 or weigh less than 60kg to run a marathon. A look at the myriad shapes, sizes and ages of finishers of any marathon proves that. Providing you are willing to commit the time to training, have no pre-existing medical condition that precludes it and plan your training carefully, there's no reason why you shouldn't do a marathon, whatever your current fitness level, weight or age. But you have to be realistic about what you can achieve. You may have to walk some of the way, or aim to finish, rather than worrying about times. Training for a marathon is time- and energy-consuming. Every runner crossing the finish line – be it in just over two hours or just over five – needs two things: preparation and determination.

The time you need to train for a marathon depends on where you are now. I would never recommend allowing less than 12 weeks, even if you're very fit; and if you're just starting, you'll need at least six months to get race ready. For more information see my book *Marathon & Half Marathon: From Start to Finish*.

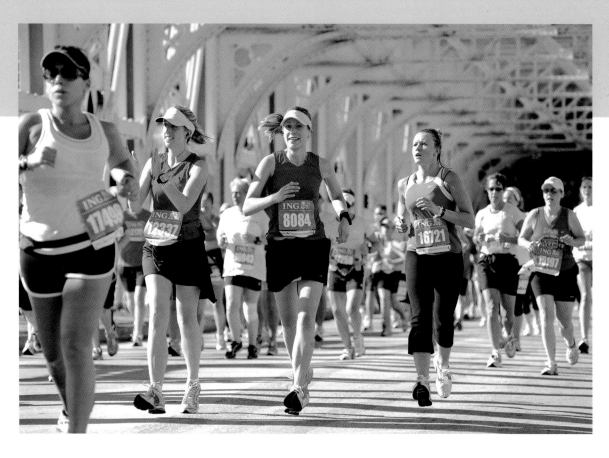

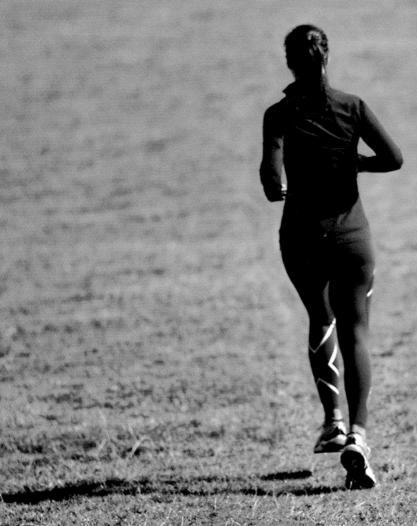

Safe and sound

Going solo
Personal safety when running alone

Running in local woodland, I was once confronted by the sight of a man emerging with an axe. I practically fell down with shock until I realised he was doing some tree clearing. It made an amusing story afterwards, but it also made me reflect on how vulnerable we can be when running alone.

It's always safer to run with someone else – even your dog – than to run alone, but if you like to go solo or there isn't anyone to run with, you need to be discerning about where and when you go and take a few sensible precautions. Here are some strategies I consider important:

- Use routes that you are familiar with, so there's no risk of getting lost or ending up in dodgy areas.
- Try to run where there will be other people – perhaps dog walkers or cyclists – and at times when there are more people around.
- Carry a personal alarm and make sure it is accessible, not tucked away in your rucksack.
- If you're running off the beaten track, ensure that you know where the nearest road or point of civilisation is.
- If you're running after dark, wear a woolly hat with your hair tucked inside and a loose top or jacket so that you could pass for male or female at first glance.
- Have no qualms about turning back or taking a different route if your original plan means going past someone or something you don't feel happy about. If a car pulls up next to you, it's most likely they want to ask directions, but at night or if there aren't many people around, it's best not to take a chance and carry on running.
- Don't wear headphones. If you're running alone, it's important that you stay aware and alert. This applies as much to traffic as it does to the risk of someone following you.

- Always tell someone where you're going and how long you think you'll be. If there's no one home, leave a note or send a text.
- On long runs and off-road routes, carry a mobile phone, in case you run into difficulties. Some cash can also be handy.
- Vary your routes – don't always run your 10km loop on Wednesday mornings. It's just possible that someone unsavoury may take note of the fact that you are always in a particular place at that time, and act upon it.

Please don't be put off running alone – most of the above measures are common sense, and would apply equally to taking the dog for a walk. The important thing is always to be aware of your surroundings and to avoid taking unnecessary risks. You may consider taking a self-defence class to improve your knowledge of what to do should you ever find yourself in a threatening situation.

Dealing with dogs

From over-protective guard dogs chasing you off their property to over-enthusiastic dogs almost tripping you over, other people's dogs can be the bane of a runner's life. Try to pass dogs that are off-lead at a walk, rather than a run. Most dogs don't mean any harm – they just get excited because you are running and they like running too. A dog may react negatively if it thinks you are trespassing or threatening its owner, so give properties where dogs are running free a wide berth and don't run between a dog and its owner. Don't stare directly at a dog if it is growling at you; show that you aren't a threat by looking away and backing off.

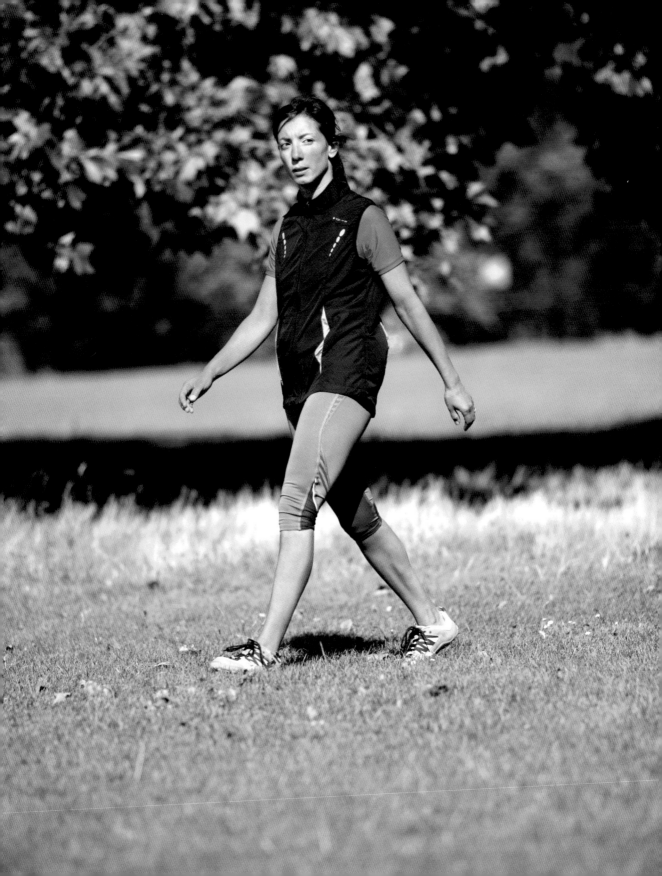

Damage limitation
How to deal with injuries

Even if you do everything right in terms of your training, recovery and nutrition, there's no guarantee that you won't get injured. How you deal with the early signs of a problem can make a big difference to how long you're sidelined for. Ignoring a niggle is a surefire way of allowing it to develop into something more serious. Yet this is something that runners do all the time. It's as if it's quite normal to run with a sore knee or a throbbing ankle. But it isn't!

The key is distinguishing between 'good' pain – generalised soreness, which says you worked hard and successfully overloaded the body – and 'bad' pain, which says you did something too hard, for too long, or did it badly. This pain doesn't quickly ease off when you run but, instead, it gets worse or causes you to alter how you run to avoid stressing the area further.

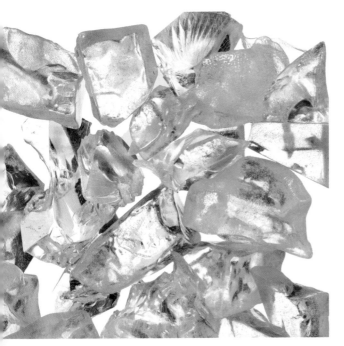

Chronic or acute?

There are two categories of injury – 'acute' and 'chronic'.

Acute injuries happen suddenly, like twisting your ankle or pulling a hamstring. (Joint injuries are called sprains; muscular injuries are known as strains, pulls or tears). You almost certainly won't be able to continue running, and you should follow the RICE protocol (see opposite) as soon as possible. Taking the appropriate measures in the first 48 hours can help to reduce the severity of the injury.

Chronic injuries, on the other hand, creep up on you, perhaps starting as a faint niggle and only gradually worsening. These are far more common among runners – problems such as plantar fasciitis, runner's knee and iliotibial band friction syndrome fit into this category. Chronic injuries are generally a result of overuse (doing too much training overall or increasing volume too quickly) or misuse (training errors, such as running in the wrong shoes or poor biomechanics). The R and I of RICE (see opposite) can help to dampen down inflammation and alleviate pain, as can anti-inflammatories. Sports massage or self-massage can help to get rid of waste products created by healing and gently stretch out scar tissue. But what's really important is finding out what the problem is, and what caused it, so you can prevent it happening again. Looking back through your training journal can be helpful in identifying potential triggers. Did you note down when you were first aware of a niggle in that area? Had your mileage gone up suddenly?

The RICE protocol

Follow the RICE protocol for 48 hours when dealing with acute injuries. Resist the temptation to take anti-inflammatory painkillers (non anti-inflammatory painkillers, like paracetamol, are fine) during this time, when the body is undergoing its own 'inflammatory response' to kickstart the healing process. Also avoid massage and heat.

R is for Rest Take stress off the injured part as soon as possible; don't keep 'testing' it to see if it feels better.

I is for Ice Apply ice to the injured area for eight minutes every couple of hours to reduce blood flow and inflammation. Do not put ice directly on your skin – wrap a damp tea towel around a liquid ice pack, ice cubes or frozen peas. Even cold water is beneficial, if you don't have immediate access to ice.

C is for Compression A crepe bandage or compression sleeve will help reduce swelling. It also serves to hold the ice pack in place.

E is for Elevation Try to raise the injured area to promote blood flow away from the injury towards the heart.

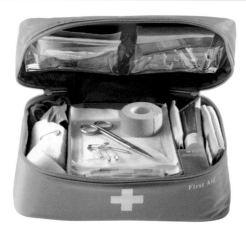

Get moving

While it's important to allow time for the injury, whether chronic or acute, to settle, you should aim to introduce some gentle movement again as soon as possible after the first 48 hours. Restoring mobility is an important part of rehabilitation, but only use a range of motion that is pain-free – even if that is just bending and straightening your knee or circling your ankle. Gradually increase the range and intensity of movement, as far as pain allows, and don't start running until you can do so comfortably. Cross-training activities are invaluable, helping maintain your fitness without over-stressing the healing area (see p. 84).

Consult the experts

If the problem isn't improving after a few days of proactive measures – or if it comes back within days of getting going again – seek a diagnosis. If you continue to run with pain, other body parts will compensate and your problems may multiply. The sooner you know what you're dealing with, the sooner you can take steps to heal your injury and prevent it recurring. Research published in the *Archives of Internal Medicine* found that only around half of all running injuries are new trouble areas; the other half are recurrences of previous problems. This demonstrates how important it is to get to the root of injuries, rather than just dealing with the symptoms.

This book does not cover the symptoms or treatment of running-related injuries (for a detailed look at running injuries, see my book *Running Well*, co-written with leading physiotherapist, Sarah Connors). Self diagnosis can be risky, because even if it is correct, you may not know the best form of rehabilitation or, more importantly, why you got injured in the first place. It isn't as simple as a specific injury always being caused by the same factor – any injury can have a number of possible causes. And just because it hurts in location A, it doesn't mean that the cause isn't location B; weak hips are often the culprit behind runner's knee,

Achilles tendinitis, and iliotibial-band syndrome, according to the University of Calgary's Running Injury Clinic.

Who should you see for advice? In theory, your GP should be your first port of call when injury strikes, but my own experiences (and those of many runners) suggest that you need to be very lucky to have a doctor who understands running – how important it is to you, how telling you to give it up isn't helpful and how best to address running-related injuries. Ideally, you'll be referred to a physiotherapist or other sports medicine professional, but the chances are you'll wait a long time before you get an appointment. If that's the case, you may be better off going straight to an expert. To help find the sports medicine expert best suited to your needs, here's the lowdown on what they all do. Try to get a recommendation from someone locally – your local running store or club:

Podiatrist

A podiatrist is a kind of foot doctor, but that doesn't mean they only deal with black toenails and heel pain. Podiatists also look at the effect of footstrike on the body's mechanics and are a good point of contact for running gait-related problems. This is who you need to see if you're advised to have orthotics made.

Physiotherapist

A physiotherapist uses manual manipulation, such as deep-tissue massage and assisted stretching, along with treatment aids, such as ultrasound, to address existing soft-tissue injuries or help prevent them. A physiotherapist will usually give you home exercises or stretches to do.

Chiropractor

Chiropractors are concerned with the alignment of bones and the effect alignment has on the spine, the nervous system and the joints. They use high-speed 'adjustments' to restore normal function and movement to a problem area. A gentler form, known as McTimoney chiropractic, doesn't manipulate bones into place, but uses vibration to encourage the bones to realign themselves.

Osteopath

Osteopaths work with their hands using a variety of treatments to deal with bone and joint problems (especially back pain). These may include soft-tissue techniques, rhythmic passive joint mobilisation or short, sharp 'thrust' techniques designed to improve mobility and the range of joint movement (similar to a chiropractor).

Sports massage therapist

Sports massage therapists are best for general tightness, aches and pains. They are not qualified to diagnose injuries, although they are able to iron out and warn you about areas that feel very tight or knotted, which can be injuries waiting to happen.

Getting the most from your sports medicine specialist

- **Show and tell** Take your training diary with you to help you be precise when you explain what led up to the injury.
- **Take notes** You might not remember that it was your piriformis in spasm or a weak quadratus lumborum at the root of your problem, once you've left the clinic.

Are you injury prone?

I'm not talking about having two left feet, but about your personality. Research suggests that runners who are aggressive, tense and compulsive have a higher risk of injury because they refuse to listen to the early warning signs of an injury and push themselves through pain and fatigue. These 'type-A' individuals lose twice as much training time when injury occurs. It's also been found that injury occurrence is higher when people are stressed or sleep-deprived.

- **Ask for diagrams** If you are given exercises to do, make sure you know exactly how to do them. Ask the practitioner to write down how many and how often and, ideally, to draw stick drawings showing how to perform them.
- **See a soulmate** If possible, find a specialist who is either a runner or who treats runners. This makes such a difference, as they are likely to keep abreast of the latest techniques and research. If they were into swimming, they might know everything there is to know about the shoulder, but not a lot about the knee.
- **Get to the root** Your main priority is getting rid of the injury. But making sure it doesn't happen again is equally important, and that is dependent on the specialist figuring out what caused it. Make sure they tell you too.
- **Do as you are told** You've invested in someone's expertise, so follow their instructions, whether that's performing rehab exercises, refraining from running or applying ice twice a day.

Life sentence?

Some injuries, and their causes, are tricky to get on top of. But that doesn't mean that you should see the physio twice a week forever. Be wary if your treatment seems to be going on and on; by showing and telling you what you can do to help yourself, and treating the injury appropriately, your practitioner should be able to dismiss you within a few weeks. Denying you the information you need to help yourself rehabilitate is taking away your control of the situation.

Finally, try to be patient and stay positive. I'm only too aware of how frustrating it can be to not be able to run, but research suggests that having a positive attitude can help you recover faster. Focus on what you can do, rather than what you can't, and be as committed to your rehabilitation as you are to running. In all likelihood, you will be back in your running shoes sooner rather than later.

Pill popping

Non-steroidal anti-inflammatory drugs (NSAIDs) are sometimes jokingly referred to by runners as 'vitamin I', the 'I' standing for ibuprofen, one of the most common drugs in this group. NSAIDs can help reduce inflammation and relieve pain, but many runners use them to prevent muscle soreness, popping a couple of pills before heading out for a run. Research from Appalachian State University suggests that this is ineffective and could even be dangerous. The maximum safe daily dose is 1200mg, to be taken in doses of 200–400mg (there is no demonstrable benefit in taking more than 400mg at a time in relieving pain or other symptoms). Excessive use (e.g. taking the drug every day for a long period) can raise the risk of gastrointestinal bleeding or other stomach problems. It can also affect kidney function; there is some evidence to suggest a link between runners taking high levels of NSAIDs and hyponatraemia (see p.147), as well as renal failure. The best way to avoid potentially harmful side effects is to use NSAIDs only to treat, rather than prevent, muscle soreness and to stick to the recommended guidelines. Never use drugs to numb pain and allow you to run.

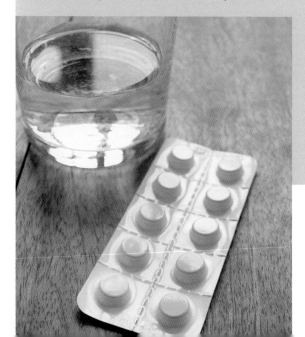

Running into trouble
Common afflictions and annoyances

From stitches and cramps to toilet crises, there are many afflictions runners have to contend with while pounding the pavements. Prevention is always better than cure, so this section addresses both for some common conditions.

Delayed onset muscle soreness (DOMS)

The problem DOMS is general soreness and muscular aches, which usually appear one or two days after unaccustomed exertion. It is caused by microtrauma – tiny tears that occur in the muscles as a result of heavy exercise.

Solution Rest or a gentle activity that doesn't exacerbate soreness is the best bet. According to *Physician and Sports Medicine*, gentle stretching and ice may help to speed recovery while anti-inflammatories can alleviate the soreness.

Prevention Don't overdo it. Increase your volume of training gradually, and space out tougher sessions.

Gastrointestinal (GI) issues

The problem GI symptoms such as nausea, vomiting, belching, bloating, heartburn, stomach cramps and diarrhoea are experienced by 20–50 per cent of athletes according to the *American Journal of Gastroenterology*. Finding the cause is a case of trial and error. It may be the timing of meals prior to a run or the food itself. The jolting movement of the body during running can also cause gastrointestinal disturbances.

Solution If you are running in an urban area, you should be able to find a public toilet. If there aren't any, most gyms or health clubs will be sympathetic to a passing runner. Or there's always the pub.

If you are somewhere rural, find a private spot slightly off the trail, but be careful of unstable ground and stinging nettles. You may want to jog up the track first to check that no one is coming the other way. Carrying some loo paper is wise if you are prone to running-induced trots, but if you're having a wee in the wild, it's kinder to the environment to forgo the loo paper.

Prevention If you always need 'to go' after a short period of running, a popular remedy is to have a cup of coffee before you leave – this usually stimulates the bowels. However, caffeine and alcohol are known stomach irritants, so try not to drink too much of either if you are prone to tummy problems. Avoid high-fibre foods just before a run, and experiment with eliminating dairy products prior to running, which may help. Another common cause of gastrointestinal upsets during running is the high sugar content of sports drinks. You may find that diluting yours drink with a little water helps to alleviate the problem.

Muscle cramp

The problem Research shows that 67 per cent of runners have experienced muscle cramp during running. It is most common in muscles that cross more than one joint; for example, the gastrocnemius muscle in the calf, which crosses the ankle and knee, and the biceps femoris, one of the hamstrings, which crosses the hip and knee. Lack of salt used to be blamed, but the more recent 'muscle fatigue' hypothesis suggests cramp or 'exercise associated muscle cramp' (EAMC) results from haphazard and involuntary muscle contractions caused by fatigue. The fatigue may be general exhaustion during long exercise, but it could also be specific to a muscle group that was overworked due to a muscular imbalance, lack of flexibility or poor biomechanics.

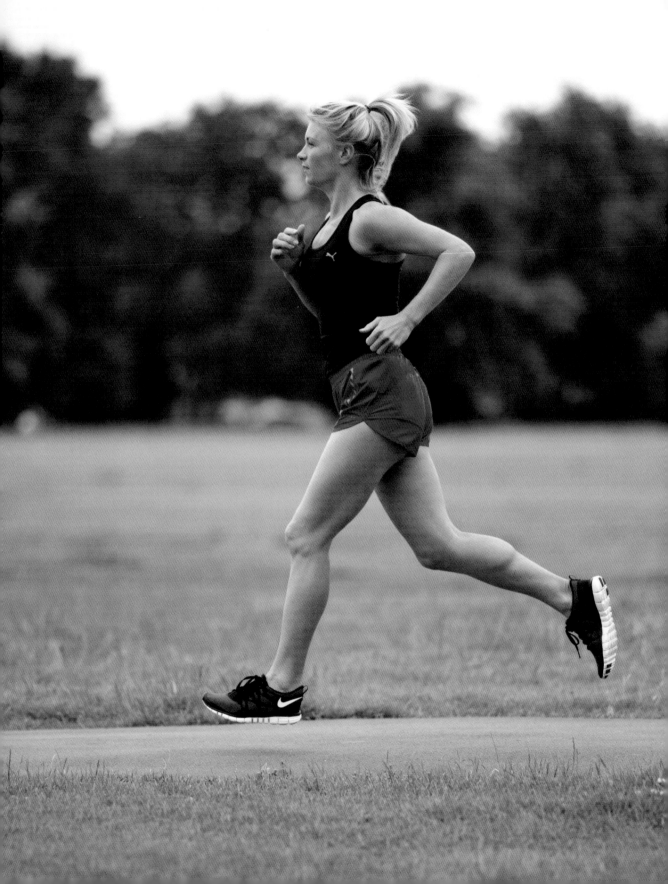

Solution Stretching the muscle is one of the best solutions, according to research at Cape Town University. It's also worth experimenting with isotonic sports drinks to remedy the problem. Research from the University of Alabama found that consuming a sports drink helped to delay the onset of EAMC in cramp-prone athletes, but 69 per cent of them did experience cramp at some point during fatigue-inducing exercise.

Prevention If cramp is a regular issue, assess your flexibility in the relevant joints and work on correcting any biomechanical faults that might be causing the problem.

Stitches

The problem Modern science still hasn't fathomed out why we get stitches, or what the science boffs call 'exercise-related transient abdominal pain' (ETAP). One study found that 69 per cent of runners had suffered a stitch in the past year. Theories abound regarding the cause, from cramping of the abdominal muscles as a result of insufficient oxygen, to irritation of the ligaments supporting the diaphragm caused by the jolting effects of running. One of the most plausible theories concerns the peritoneum, the layers of tissue that line the abdominal wall. Scientists speculate that the pain could be friction between the inner and outer layers of tissue, due to a drop in the fluid between them (so the two layers are closer together), distention of the stomach (pushing the inner layer onto the outer one) or simply a result of excess movement of the two layers. ETAP is often accompanied by shoulder-tip pain, which supports this theory, because both areas are supplied by the same nerve. Research published in the *Journal of Science and Medicine* in Sport in 2010 postulates that a stiff thoracic spine and a 'kyphotic' posture (where the upper spine is excessively hunched forward) are more commonly associated with stitches. Researchers recommend posture-corrective exercises to help the problem.

Solution Try synchronising your breathing with your footstrike when you get a stitch. This hasn't worked for me, but if I dig my fingers into the painful area and knead it, the stitch usually goes. A survey of runners found that bending forwards, stretching the painful area, contracting the abdominals and breathing deeply were other successful strategies. These all necessitate slowing down or stopping, which might in itself ease the pain.

Prevention To avoid a stitch, researchers suggest eating small amounts of food before a run, avoiding foods high in sugar and fat pre-run and steering clear of certain foods, including apples, dairy products and chocolate. What you drink may also be worth considering. A study in the International Journal of Sport Nutrition and Exercise Metabolism found that when exercisers drank either flavoured water, a sports drink, fruit juice or nothing at all, a stitch was most prevalent in those drinking fruit juice. Other preventative strategies include core stability exercises to strengthen the abdominal region and a thorough warm-up to allow for lubrication of the peritoneum. The good news is that stitches seem to ease with age.

Urinary incontinence

The problem It is the unmentionable problem, yet urinary incontinence (UI) affects as many as 50 per cent of all women, particularly after pregnancy – and it can really hamper your running. There are two types of UI –

'stress' incontinence, where a sudden movement such as jumping or a sneeze, causes you to leak urine, and 'urge' incontinence, where you get a sudden need to go, which isn't always controllable.

In both cases (but especially with stress incontinence) pelvic floor muscle strengthening or 'Kegel' exercises can help. The pelvic floor muscles – the main one of which is called the pubococcygeus – form a figure-of-eight shape around the vagina and anus. These muscles support the contents of the pelvis and abdomen and control the emptying of the bladder and bowels and the contraction of the vagina. When they become weakened, through misuse, disease or damage, they are less able to do their job properly.

Solution The first course of action is pelvic floor exercises. If done correctly, these are 90 per cent effective in stopping UI. When women say they don't work, it is often because they have done far too few to make a difference, or done them incorrectly. Be patient – one study review found that regular training for three months or more yielded the best results. Here's how to do them:

- **Step 1: locating the pelvic floor** Firstly, you need to find the muscles. To do this, imagine you need to pass wind but have to hold it in. The muscles you feel 'squeezing' around the anus are the rear of the pelvic floor muscles. Now imagine you need a wee, but have to stop yourself going. The muscles you feel tightening to stop the flow of urine are the front end of the pelvic floor muscles. You may find that sucking your thumb while pulling up your pelvic floor muscles helps to get a good contraction. It's fine to try to locate the muscles when you are actually on the loo, if you find this easier, but don't do it regularly, as you may irritate your bladder.
- **Step 2: contracting the pelvic floor** To strengthen the muscles, start to 'pull them up' from the back to the front. Contract the muscles slowly and hold the squeeze (build up to ten seconds), then relax for a few seconds before repeating. Aim for five pull-ups to begin with, then gradually increase to 8–12

repetitions. Don't hold your breath while you are doing these exercises. Next, pull the muscles up quickly and tightly, and then relax them immediately – the same movement, but much faster. Again, start with doing these five times and increase the number gradually (up to 8–12 times).

You should exercise your pelvic floor three times a day. The easiest position is sitting down or standing, with your legs slightly apart, but once you get familiar with the exercises, you will be able to do them in any position.

In addition to doing pelvic floor exercises, make sure you always visit the loo last thing before you leave to go running. And don't be tempted to avoid drinking to reduce your chances of an incontinent episode. Keep coffee, caffeinated drinks (remember, some sports drinks contain caffeine) and alcohol to a minimum – these can all exacerbate the problem.

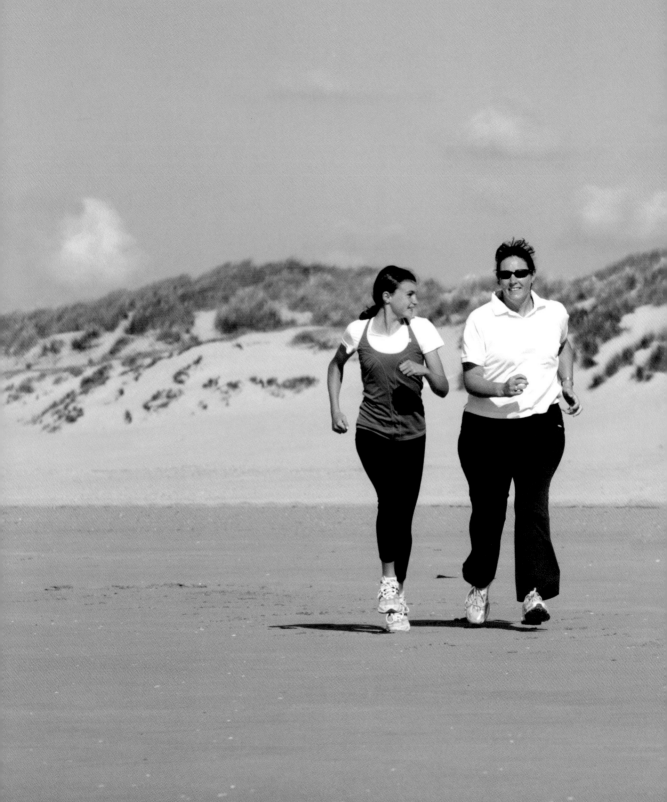

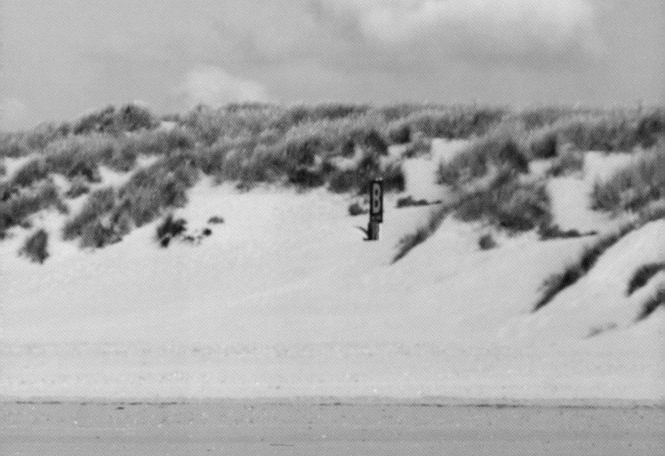

Run for life

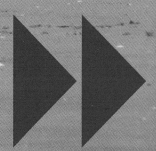

Child's play
Encouraging kids to run

Children don't need to be told to run – they do it instinctively. Whether they are chasing a ball, or each other, running is part of their everyday play. Or at least, it used to be. But with an ever-increasing focus on computer games and social networking – not to mention TV – kids are becoming more sedentary than ever before. So it's no surprise that one in three children in the UK between 2 and 15 years of age is overweight or obese. You can't force your kids to go outside and run (doing so will probably put them off for life), but you can create opportunities for running which are fun and varied – and you can educate them about how good running is for them. A review study from the University of Georgia concluded that regular exercise can enhance children's brain function and development, while other research shows that children with the highest physical activity levels at the age of five are least likely to be overweight at 8 and 11 years of age. The pre-teen years are an important time for developing bone mass, particularly in girls; research suggests that the greatest increases in bone mineral density take place when weight-bearing exercise, like running, is started in the five years prior to the onset of their periods.

Fun running

As a runner, you are already providing an excellent role model for your children, but what else can you do to encourage them to follow in your footsteps? A continuous run, of the sort you probably do, isn't likely to appeal to younger ones. Simple games like tag and stuck-in-the-mud work really well, or you could get children into groups and try relays or team races. With young children, don't focus on specific distances or times, and when they stop and start, let them – it's their way of balancing effort with recovery. Orienteering is another great way to get the whole family involved in running (see 'Girls' talk', p. 187).

The usual injury prevention rules apply to children – from the importance of warming up to not building up time or distance too quickly and taking sufficient rest days. It's wise to ensure that children run on softer surfaces wherever possible, such as level grass. Kids can't regulate body temperature as well as adults, so monitor them for signs of overheating – always have water at hand and encourage them to drink when thirsty.

What if your child does want to come for 'a run' with you? It's difficult to say whether this is appropriate because children differ widely in their physical development and fitness level for their age. The International Federation of Athletic Federations (IAAF) offers guidelines on what distances are appropriate for different age groups, but these only start at nine years old (see opposite). That doesn't mean a younger child cannot go for a run, but how far and how fast has to be guided by them, not you. It's best to limit your outings together to one or two short runs a week maximum – partly because that's probably enough 'straight' running for them, but also because if their presence hampers your training, you might resent it, which could make the experience less enjoyable for you both. IAAF guidelines recommend that children under 14 do not exceed three runs a week.

Jack of all trades

It is also important to bear in mind any other physical activity your child is doing. Experts stress the importance of kids engaging in a range of sports and activities in their formative years – anything from swimming to gymnastics, martial arts to dancing – but a budding young athlete could easily end up doing an excessive amount of training, so keep an eye on their overall physical activity. 'A little bit of everything' is better than too much of one activity, at least in the pre-teen years; most athletics organisations don't recommend that children specialise in a specific sport until they reach 12 or 13. This is partly to do with physical development – over-stressing the same muscle groups and bones repeatedly is more likely to result in injury or growth problems, as well as creating imbalances – but it's also psychological. Over-enthusiastic coaches or parents can pile on pressure or expectation, leading children to burn out or give up.

If you can encourage, rather than insist, support, rather than push and make running fun and rewarding, you may just be setting your son or daughter on the path to a healthier, fitter and longer life.

Kids' running checklist

Make sure you can say yes to all five of the following statements:

✓ She/he is having fun.
✓ She/he wants to run.
✓ She/he is setting the pace and taking breaks where necessary.
✓ She/he has the energy and interest to do other non-running activities.
✓ She/he isn't getting aches or pains from running.

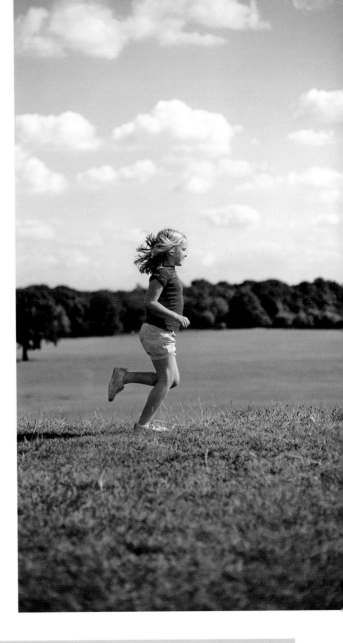

Age (in years)	Maximum distance per session/race	Maximum weekly training distance
Under 9	3km	6km
9–11	5km	10km
12–14	10km	20km
15–16	Half marathon (21.1km)	40km

Guidelines from the International Association of Athletics Federations (IAAF)

Teenage kicks
Getting young girls active

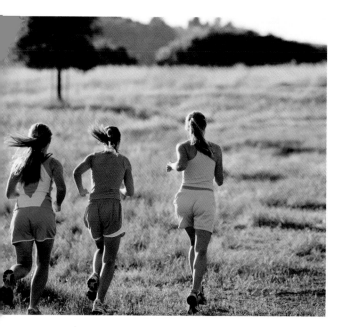

Bodily changes, self-consciousness and a burgeoning interest in other things (namely, social networking and boys) make teenage girls one of the hardest groups to attract to, or keep, running. A study in the *Journal of Sports Medicine and Physical Fitness* found that girls aged 12–15 who were least active said they 'didn't like' physical activity and that they 'weren't any good at sport'. This highlights a key problem: teenage girls' experience and perception of physical activity.

For too long, physical activity within schools has meant sport. Sport means competition – winners and losers. One survey of teenage girls found that a negative experience of PE was the main factor putting them off physical activity. While non-competitive activities, such as dance and martial arts, are beginning to appear on the curriculum – running still seems to be viewed as a sport, rather than as a form of exercise. The same problem exists within athletics clubs – rather than welcoming runners of all abilities, the bias is all too often towards those with natural talent and a desire to develop it.

A study in the *Journal of Sport Behaviour* found that teenage girls' main motivation for exercise was to have fun and make friends. If running fails to tick those boxes, it's likely that they won't stick with it. While fun and social reasons might draw teenage girls towards physical activity, a lack of confidence in or embarrassment about their physical ability can drive them away from it. The earlier a girl decides she's 'no good' at sport, the more likely she is to avoid it, compromising her development of sporting skills and setting up a self-fulfilling prophecy.

How can we get teenage girls more active? You're already taking one of the most powerful steps by being active yourself: the *Journal of Sport Behaviour* found that girls were more likely to take exercise if their mothers did. Running together could provide a great bonding opportunity. You could set a shared goal, such as training for a women-only event like one of the UK-wide Race for Life 5km series. Female-only groups, such as those run by Women on the Run, are another great option. The emphasis is on taking part, having fun and getting fit, rather than winning races and scoring points.

A healthy perspective

Whether running during adolescence is a continuation of an active childhood or a new challenge, it's a time when there are many mental and physical benefits to be gained.

A quarter of adult bone mass is acquired between the ages of 12 and 14, and weight-bearing activity helps to optimise this. It's also a healthy way to maintain or achieve an appropriate weight. A 2007 study found that when adolescent girls tried to lose weight, they employed unhealthy techniques (like restricting energy intake and bingeing) and did not include physical activity. Over a five-year period this led to a rise in body mass index (BMI) and an increase in disordered eating (see p. 191).

Research suggests that active teenagers have a more positive body image than their non-active peers. With scoiety's continuing obsession with appearance, focusing the mind on what the body can do, rather than what it looks like can lead to greater body satisfaction and self-esteem. German research in the journal *Psychology & Health* in 2009 found that even a single bout of exercise made young women feel better about themselves; they felt slightly slimmer and more satisfied with their bodies after exercising compared to spending the same time reading a newspaper. As with adults, running can also help teenagers deal with stress and combat depression.

Getting teenagers running may even improve their exam results. Research from the University of Gothenburg found that improving aerobic fitness between the ages of 15 and 18 enhances cognitive performance, particularly logical thinking and verbal understanding.

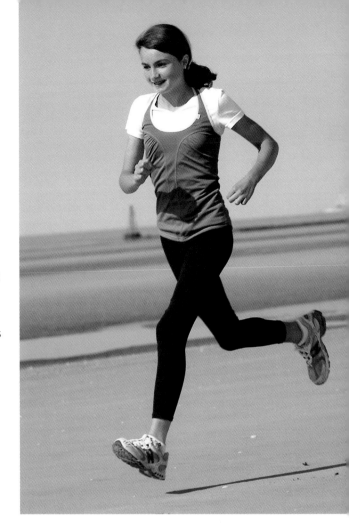

Teenage tips

- Make sure they are wearing kit they feel attractive in. One study found that teenage girls worry about appearing 'sweaty' and 'muscular', rather than 'attractive' and 'feminine' when exercising. A longer-fitting top that skims the hips works well for those who are self-conscious about their bottoms.
- Growing girls need adequate bust support (see p. 122).
- Encourage them not to 'cover up' with too many layers or they risk overheating.
- Make sure they eat adequate calcium to support bone growth (see p. 142).
- Watch for signs of disordered eating, over-training or excessive fatigue.
- If their periods have started, but then become absent after taking up running, seek advice (see p. 191).

> "
> As the kids get older they can enjoy running with you. If they think running is boring, you could try looking for an orienteering event. Choose one of the shortest courses with really easy map reading and run together, encouraging your child to be the first to spot the markers.
>
> *Elly*

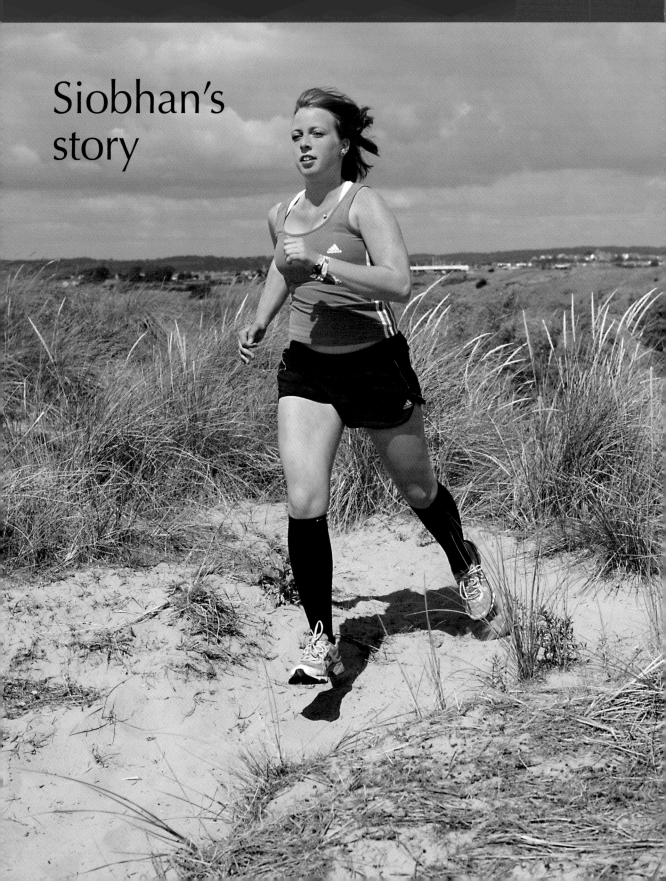

Siobhan's
story

'I felt fit, focused and ready for the challenge of university'

"

My parents took up running when I was in my mid-teens, so I was dragged along to road races on cold Sunday mornings to watch them. I thought they were mad; it looked tough, tiring and, to make matters worse, it was an all-weather sport!

Inevitably, it wasn't long before I was collared into having a go myself. It was a 2km fun run, but it felt like a marathon. The rain poured down at a torrential rate, and the wind was so strong it blew me back two steps for each one I took forwards. I didn't go again.

That was until I came face-to-face with my A Level exams and the prospect of going to university. Weighed down by the stress of my academic work, I accepted my parents' invitation to go for a run. This time, I loved it. I went out again and again, and managed to run a little further each time. The first time I did a whole run without stopping to walk was so inspiring – I finally felt like I was getting to know my body.

Each time I felt the stress building, I put on my trainers and hit the road. It cleared my head, gave me energy and a fresh motivation to tackle the revision books when I got back. Needless to say, my friends thought I was mad, but while they were worrying about whether or not they would get the grades, I felt confident.

When I got to university, I joined the athletics club and my running improved at a phenomenal rate. But, more than that, I met like-minded people who, even though they were all looking to get something different from the sport, all wanted to run. I felt fit, focused and ready to face every challenge the new world of university threw at me.

During my time at uni, I've seen many people join the athletics club and develop a passion for running, and there are two things that I've noticed about all of them. The first is that everyone who comes along confesses that they 'can't' run; there is no such thing as being unable to run, it's just a question of learning how to suit your body to it. Secondly, everyone who takes it up vows they'll never go back to a lazy lifestyle. So if you're sat there reading this book and wondering whether you really can run, you've already taken your first step by considering it. Your second step is to get out there on the road: whether you run 20 metres or 20 minutes, it will be the start of something great!

"

The time of the month
Running and the menstrual cycle

Does your monthly cycle affect your running performance? Menstruation has a vastly different effect on different women. Some barely notice their periods, while others struggle with heavy bleeding and cramps. If it's not the period itself, premenstrual syndrome (PMS) can interfere with your running. The American College of Obstetricians and Gynaecologists estimates that 85 per cent of menstruating women suffer from at least one symptom of PMS, whether physical or mental. Common psychological symptoms include appetite changes, mood swings and depression, while physical effects range from tender breasts to backache, bloating and water retention.

> I always make myself run on the first day of my period – it makes me feel so much better.
>
> Jackie

Combating PMS and period pain

Can exercise help? In terms of curbing the severity of PMS symptoms, the answer appears to be yes. A study from Shiraz University in Iran found that three hours of exercise per week for 12 weeks reduced physical and psychological premenstrual symptoms, while research from Duke University in Durham, North Carolina found that aerobic exercise (like running) was more effective in mitigating symptoms than anaerobic exercise, like strength training.

But the evidence with regard to period pain is less clear cut. After quizzing 650 18–25-year-olds on their activity levels and menstrual cycle experience, a 2009 Birmingham University study proclaimed that the evidence that exercise could help to ease menstrual cramps was no more than anecdotal. There were no significant differences in activity level between the 72 per cent who didn't suffer pain and the 28 per cent who suffered moderate to severe pain. However, research by Arkansas University found that in women over 30 years old, there was less cramping, breast tenderness and bloating in active women compared to their non-active peers. Researchers suggest that exercise may help by increasing levels of endorphin – the body's 'feel-good' hormone – as well as inhibiting prostaglandins, the hormone-like substances that make nerves more sensitive.

Another issue concerns the effects of fluctuating hormones on women's joint stability. Some trials have shown that sportswomen tend to suffer more ligament injuries – particularly the anterior cruciate ligament (ACL) in the knee – around ovulation (mid-cycle), due to hormones causing increased joint laxity and decreased 'stiffness'

No periods?

An absence of periods in any pre-menopausal woman should not be ignored, but is of particular concern in teenage girls and young women.

In very active women, the most common cause is a low energy intake – not taking in enough calories to match energy expenditure. This can be an early warning sign of disordered eating or of excessive exercise to facilitate weight loss. There is also a direct correlation between the duration of amenorrhoea (an absence of periods for three months or more) and a reduction in bone mineral density. Given the importance of the early teenage years in forming bone mass, this is not a time this process should be compromised. One study found 52 per cent of women with osteoporosis in adulthood had suffered menstrual disorders in adolescence.

Disordered eating and amenorrhoea can occur independently of one another, but a condition known as the 'female athlete triad' has been identified, in which amenorrhoea is accompanied by disordered eating and low bone mass. The American College of Sports Medicine recommends that female athletes (or more active females) diagnosed with one of the conditions should be screened for the other two.

of the muscles and tendons. Studies suggest that the contraceptive pill can reduce this risk, but that's not an option for everyone. ACL injuries tend to be a result of multi-directional sports like netball, skiing and tennis so don't be unduly concerned – runners are more at risk of 'overuse' injuries than acute ligament injuries.

How to minimise the impact of your menstrual cycle on your training

1. Fuel your body. You need an extra 150–220 calories in the lead-up to a period, due to a hike in metabolic rate. Don't deny yourself and risk falling short of energy.
2. Make sure you have a supportive and comfortable sports bra to wear in your pre-menstrual phase, when your breasts may be as much as a size bigger.
3. Take NSAID painkillers at the first hint of menstrual cramp – this appears to be more effective than waiting for the ache to take hold.
4. Try scheduling your key sessions (races, or important training runs) for the second half of your menstrual cycle. One study found that women performing the same workout between days five and seven (where day one is the first day of your period) and then again between days 19 and 21 found the early cycle workout harder; interestingly, they also burned a lower proportion of fat.
5. Consider complementary health approaches to reducing period pain and PMS symptoms. Omega-3-rich foods, such as oily fish, are believed to dampen down inflammation in the body, while evening primrose oil can alleviate breast soreness.
6. Keep note of your menstrual cycle in your training journal to see if there is a pattern of energy highs and lows or changes in your performance.

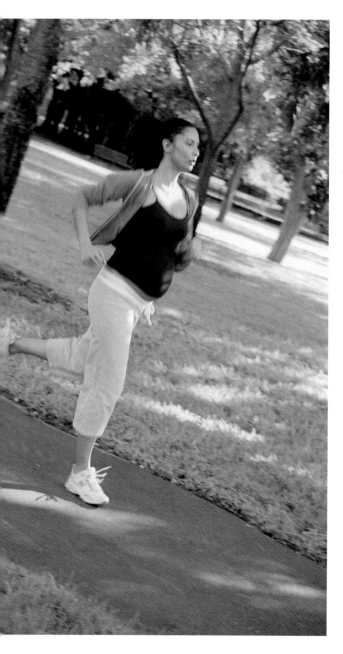

If running is a big part of your life when you fall pregnant, you may be concerned about whether you can continue running without putting your baby or yourself at risk. There's plenty of evidence that women can run during pregnancy – and that there are many benefits to be gained from doing so – but it is very much a personal choice, because women's experiences of pregnancy differ so greatly.

The benefits of being fit during pregnancy are so compelling that the American College of Obstetricians and Gynaecologists (ACOG) now recommends that even expectant mothers who have been previously sedentary should begin exercise. ACOG guidelines state that all pregnant women (in the absence of either medical or obstetric complications) should do 30 minutes or more of moderate exercise a day on most, if not all, days of the week at 60–90 per cent of their maximum heart rate, i.e. the same guidelines as for non-pregnant women.

However, ACOG categorises running as an activity that is safe for women to do if they were already doing it prior to pregnancy. It states: 'If you were a runner before you became pregnant, you often can keep running during pregnancy, although you may have to modify your routine.' If you aren't already running, now is not the time to start, but make sure you include some physical activity in your weekly routine.

Benefits of running during pregnancy

The latest research shows a range of benefits from exercise during pregnancy from a lower incidence of gestational diabetes, maternal hypertension and pre-eclampsia to less pregnancy weight gain, fewer birth complications and a lower chance of premature delivery. There are also important mental benefits. The University of Texas found that physical activity could improve self-esteem and reduce symptoms of anxiety and depression.

Even your baby benefits: in a study from the University of Geneva, the growing foetuses of active mothers had a lower fat mass and displayed improved stress tolerance, while a study in the *Journal of Clinical Endocrinology & Metabolism* found that regular moderate-intensity aerobic exercise led to a modest reduction in birth weight, which reduces the likelihood of childhood obesity. Babies born to mothers who exercised at least three times a week during pregnancy have also been found to be more alert and less fussy in their first few days.

Exercise can be helpful in combating some of the more dispiriting side effects of pregnancy – from muscle cramps to nausea and back pain. Although there is no scientific evidence to show that active women have easier births, it is likely that they can deal with labour and recover from the experience of childbirth better, as they are stronger and fitter.

Key concerns

Traditionally, the three major concerns about exercise during pregnancy have been foetal hypoxia (lack of oxygen), foetal hypoglycaemia (lack of glucose) and a potentially detrimental rise in foetal temperature. Plus, there is always a small risk of a 'trauma' injury, in which you fall over or have some kind of collision that harms the baby. But research suggests such fears are unfounded, as long as exercise is done moderately and sensibly.

A 2010 study in the *British Journal of Sports Medicine* found there was no detrimental effect on foetal wellbeing in elite pregnant runners during the second trimester, even when they ran at 90 per cent of their maximum heart rate. (Above 90 per cent, there were signs of increased heart rate in the foetus and reduced blood flow to the uterus, although these normalised when exercise ceased.)

Reassuringly, even during such intense activity, it's highly unlikely that you'd compromise your baby's wellbeing. Similarly, a study from Case Western Reserve University in Cleveland, Ohio, found that while the delivery of oxygen and glucose to the foetus may be reduced slightly during exercise, it is probable that regular bouts of sustained exercise may improve oxygen and fuel delivery at rest.

Regarding the final factor, research has not found any instances where maternal temperature has led to foetal abnormalities in humans. Avoiding exercise in hot, humid conditions (or even a hot indoor environment), as well as overlong exercise sessions, will minimise the risk. It's also vitally important to stay well hydrated.

How your body changes

The most obvious changes are weight gain and a growing bump, but many other physiological and musculoskeletal changes occur during pregnancy. The average weight gain during pregnancy is 2 stone (12.7kg); half is the foetus, plus the uterus and its contents, while the rest comes

> "
> The biggest challenges to getting back into running after the birth of my daughter were breastfeeding and sleep deprivation! I tried to get back to running 11 weeks after the birth, but trying to time feeds and runs so that I wasn't uncomfortable was tricky and, in retrospect, I probably should have left it until at least four months.
>
> Clare
> "

> *Since having Mollie, I have improved all my race times from 5km to marathon. Time for training is more precious, so has to be used wisely. And there's nothing like the thought of her face at the end of a race to make me run faster!*
>
> Emma

from increased body fat and fluid, including breast tissue. The extra weight puts more stress on your joints, which means you might need to scale back your usual routine. The majority of weight gained is stored at the front of the body, which alters your centre of gravity – to compensate, the pelvis tilts forward and the lordosis (the curve in the lower back) increases, which often causes backache.

A hormone called relaxin is secreted during pregnancy, which softens the body's ligaments (particularly those around the back and pelvis) in preparation for delivery. Relaxin levels are higher in second or subsequent pregnancies, and markedly higher in women with multiple pregnancies. Later on in pregnancy, the instability of the joints caused by ligament laxity can make weight-bearing exercise like running more risky in terms of musculoskeletal injuries. Aqua jogging (see p. 86) could be a good alternative.

Physiologically, some of the effects of pregnancy are remarkably similar to those of training. Blood volume increases by as much as 35 per cent, while stroke volume and cardiac output both rise (in the final trimester, stroke volume begins to decline again and can, combined with the increased blood volume, cause blood to pool in the limbs, leading to varicose veins). Resting heart rate rises by 15–20bpm, which means any given level of effort during exercise will feel harder than previously. Higher levels of progesterone can increase ventilation, so that you breathe more quickly and deeply.

Exercise dos and don'ts

Here are my dos and don'ts for making exercise safe, comfortable and enjoyable during pregnancy:

Do:
- inform your doctor of your intention to run and ask whether they have reason to advise you otherwise.
- wear clothing that keeps you cool – layers help you to regulate body temperature.
- wear a supportive sports bra and footwear
- empty your bladder before exercise.
- leave a couple of hours after a meal before running
- drink plenty of water.
- run on even ground or a treadmill to reduce the risk of falling or twisting an ankle.
- consider wearing a maternity belt or Lycra shorts to support your bump.
- judge intensity by the talk test (see p. 67) – you should be able to converse without too much difficulty.
- be careful when stretching – your joints will be hypermobile (less 'stable' than usual).

Do not:
- exercise to lose weight.
- exercise until fatigued.
- have time or distance goals – listen to your body.
- exercise in excessively hot or humid conditions.
- run on an empty stomach – have a meal two to three hours before you run or a carbohydrate snack 30–60 minutes before; or carry a sports drink with you.
- exercise lying on your back after the first three months; that includes stretching.

Warning signs

Stop exercising and get medical help if you experience any of these symptoms as a result of exercise:

- Vaginal bleeding
- Dizziness or feeling faint
- Increased shortness of breath
- Chest pain
- Headache
- Muscle weakness
- Calf pain or swelling
- Uterine contractions
- Decreased foetal movement
- Fluid leaking from the vagina

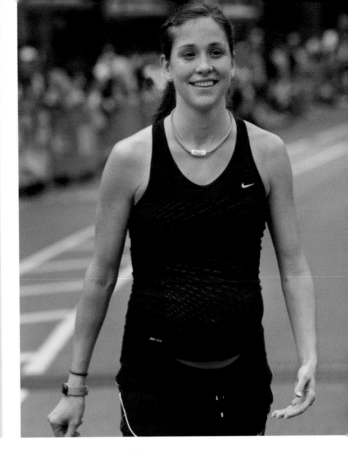

- skimp on calories; an additional 300 calories a day are needed after the first trimester.
- exercise if you have a cold, fever or infection.
- run too far from home or a reliable source of help, just in case you should start to feel unwell or something should happen; using a treadmill or running in smaller loops close to home is wise, in case you get tired or need the loo.

Contraindications for running during pregnancy

Do not run during pregnancy without medical advice if:

- you are pregnant with twins or multiple babies.
- you have had miscarriages or premature births.
- you have hypertension (high blood pressure – pregnancy-induced or otherwise).
- you have experienced bleeding.
- you feel any pain or discomfort when running.
- you don't feel confident about running

After the baby

Just as running during pregnancy is a personal choice, so is deciding when to return to it after your baby is born. Doctors often recommend waiting six weeks before doing any aerobic exercise; but some women run within days of giving birth, while for others, its weeks or months before they feel ready. Listen to your body and only do what feels right. It's advisable to try to do some exercise – even gentle walking – as soon as you feel able. A University of Michigan study found that women who were physically active after childbirth tended to feel happier and adapted better to motherhood. They also reported greater confidence about being a mum. In other research, active women were found to be at a lower risk of postnatal depression than non-active women.

Exercise can also give you a bit of much-needed 'me' time in the early months, when practically every waking minute is devoted to your baby.

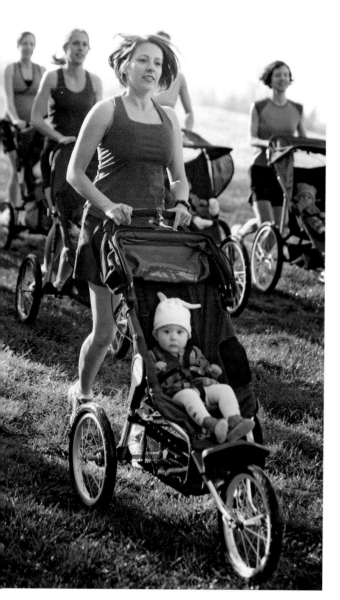

This opportunity to be yourself is one of the most frequently cited motivators for getting back to running in motherhood.

How to make a successful return to running

- Be patient. Start with walking and try very short bouts of running to see how it feels. Progress with a walk–run programme (see p. 63), gradually increasing the running bouts, as and when you can.
- Consider visiting an osteopath or chiropractor for a check-up before starting post-pregnancy exercise. Pregnancy can often tilt or twist the pelvis slightly, or affect the sacroiliac joint, which may cause back and lower-limb problems once you start running again.
- Build frequency and duration before thinking about increasing the intensity of your running.
- Don't be tempted to set yourself goals or you risk feeling stressed or disappointed that you can't do as much as you would like.
- Begin pelvic floor exercises as soon as possible (see p. 180).
- Breastfeed before activity to make running more comfortable and limit the acidity of your breast milk.
- Avoid abdominal exercises, such as sit-ups, until the opening in the abdominal wall – the linea alba – has rejoined (the rectus abdominis frequently splits down the middle during pregnancy to make way for the growing bump – a process called diastasis). Gentle core stability exercises, like drawing your navel to your spine, can help you regain abdominal strength and control.
- Make sure that your partner, friends and family understand how important it is that you get opportunities to exercise. It won't always be possible to schedule running as easily as you did pre-baby, particularly in the first few months, but take what you can!

Does pregnancy improve your performance?

There is much anecdotal evidence that women's athletic performance improves after giving birth. It's a bit of a mystery as to why this happens. It may be that the increased blood volume and accompanying red blood cell concentration enables more oxygen to be transported into the body, or that the experience of carrying extra weight for nine months acts as a training stimulus. But most experts believe that the effect is psychological. After a long enforced lay-off, you're so eager to begin running that you put in a lot of effort to get back to where you were before the birth. Or perhaps the experience of being pregnant and giving birth makes you feel empowered and mentally stronger. Or it could merely be a self-fulfilling prophecy – you read that your performance improves after having a baby and, hey presto, it does!

> I recovered quickly and easily from my first pregnancy, but things were different after my second. I don't think you can expect the same from your body after a second pregnancy, especially if they are close together. You need to build up general strength and fitness again before setting your sights on specific running goals. Be patient and don't expect miracles.
>
> Sarah C

And baby comes too...

A baby jogger or stroller offers the perfect way to run without having to fit around others' availability or feeling bad about leaving your baby. But it does take away the 'time out' factor, so it's not for everyone.

If you are considering buying one, try it out first to see whether you – and your baby – will enjoy outings on wheels. Make sure that your partner also tries it out, if they are going to be using it.

In terms of a smooth ride, look for a streamlined shape, big (but not fat) wheels and check ease of steering (a front wheel that locks when you want it to is invaluable). Some strollers even have suspension, which could be handy on less smooth surfaces. For comfort, you need the appropriate handlebar height (or one that is adjustable) and somewhere to stow your drink and other necessities while your baby will need a comfortable seat, safety harness and protection from the rain and sun. Look for models with a handbrake and safety leash for peace of

mind. You also need to consider the stroller's weight and portability. Does it fold down flat? Can you lug it up stairs? The average stroller weighs around 8–12kg and lighter models tend to be pricier. As this isn't an item you'll need for ever, you might consider buying a second-hand one – check out Ebay or ask fellow running-club members if they have one lying around.

Most manufacturers recommend that your baby should not be taken in a stroller until they are six months old, but this is erring on the safe side. The important issue is whether your baby has gained head control or not.

A race against time
Running at 40 and beyond

If you are past the first flush of youth, you may think your running days are behind you. The comment I hear most often from women who have started running in their 40s, 50s and 60s is: 'I wish I'd done this years ago.' The powerful combination of health and fitness gains, knowledge that you are 'taking action' to combat the effects of ageing and the boost to body image and self-confidence make running particularly compelling for women as they age.

If the 2009 New York marathon results are anything to go by, there's no reason to believe that you can't still be a contender as the years advance: the top three women were over 35 years old: Deratu Tulu (37), Paula Radcliffe (36) and

Lyudmila Petrova (41). But it wasn't just the front-runners – 43 per cent of all female finishers were over 40; and US statistics show that runners aged 50 plus are the fastest-growing group among marathon participants. German research shows that more than 25 per cent of 50- to 69-year-old marathon and half-marathon runners had only taken up running in the preceding five years. So if you're wondering if it's 'too late', the answer is no! You may never run as fast as you could have done at 20, but so what? You can still clock a PB and will reap enormous benefits.

Running: the anti-ageing sport

Running is one of the simplest and most effective ways of staving off the physiological effects of ageing. It reduces your risk of coronary heart disease, hypertension (high blood pressure) and diabetes, preserves bone, muscle tone and strength (preventing a steep decline in metabolic rate) and maintains co-ordination and balance. Many factors once considered to be the inevitable consequences of ageing – weight gain, reduced mobility and deteriorating cardiovascular fitness – are now believed to be caused by inactivity and lifestyle habits.

Research in 2011 from Tel Aviv University found that endurance exercise increases the number of muscle stem cells, maintaining muscle mass and enhancing the body's ability to repair muscle tissue. This is probably why older athletes are still able to perform so well. Remember the mitochondria – those aerobic energy production factories in the muscle cells? It's widely believed that mitochondrial concentration is lower in older people, but research suggests that, provided we remain active, mitochondrial

> As a veteran runner, I am not fuelled by a burning desire to beat my PB in every race, but I do want to do my best and get the most out of my body by running smart. That means warming up properly, keeping good posture and running technique, eating well and knowing my limitations. I pay attention to flexibility and core strength, have regular sports massage and never ignore niggly injuries.
>
> Joanne

activity need not decline at all. One study of 'masters' athletes (those over 60) found that in the calf muscle, the volume of mitochondria was 24–31 per cent higher than in 27-year-old runners in the same race. All had comparable finish times too.

Contrary to popular belief, there have been no studies to show a correlation between distance running and the development of osteoarthritis. Stanford University research found that runners experience less muscular and joint pain in old age than non-runners. Research from Ohio found that peri-menopausal women (average age 46) who ran 40km per week had higher bone density in the hip than non-running women, and equal bone density in the lumbar spine (although over a ten-year period, bone density declined in both groups). Weight-bearing exercise, like running, is also important in preventing the onset of osteoporosis (see p. 201).

Aerobic exercise enhances circulation and digestion, keeping your skin looking young. And while you might think that running will leave you exhausted, the opposite appears to be true. A University of Georgia study looked at 70 different trials on the effects of exercise and found that in 90 per cent of cases, sedentary people who took up regular exercise experienced less fatigue, not more.

Vigorous exercise can even help you keep your marbles for longer! Research from Madrid found that it was associated with improved mental function in older adults – especially those over 65. Even in people with existing cognitive deterioration, six months of high-intensity aerobic exercise boosted mental function, as well as benefiting fitness and body fat levels.

The best news of all? Sporty older people have a life expectancy almost four years higher than sedentary folk.

Starting in later years

The following points are worth highlighting to help older runners run safely and comfortably; as a runner in my 40s, and as a coach who has worked with many older runners, I speak from experience:

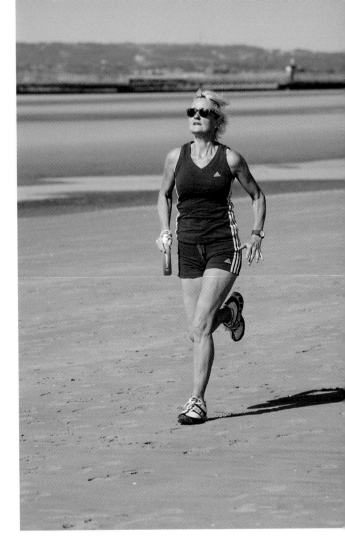

- Warm up for longer. Stiffer joints and less elasticity in muscles and other soft tissues make it even more important to warm up thoroughly before you run. Avoid sudden or extreme movements like jumps or sprints early on in your warm-up.
- Allow yourself longer to recover between tough sessions. Do this even if it means reducing the overall number of tough sessions.
- Be more vigilant about exercising in extreme temperatures. We become more prone to dehydration and heatstroke as we age, while very cold weather causes the blood vessels to constrict, putting extra strain on the heart. Dress for the conditions.

- Do some strength-training – particularly for your core stabilising muscles (see p. 101).
- Don't neglect post-run stretching – flexibility is in decline, so you need to work to hold on to what you've got. A Dutch study found that the primary cause of older runners slowing was a loss of flexibility and range of motion in the joints of the hip, knee and ankle, leading to a shorter stride length.
- Consume at least 1000mg of calcium per day. If you take a supplement, look for calcium carbonate with vitamin D because the body can absorb more calcium from this than other forms.
- Never ignore niggles. Injuries take longer to heal when we're older, so if a niggle becomes something more serious you may be sidelined for longer.

Does older mean slower?

If you don't start running until you are in your 40s or later, you have a greater potential to improve than someone who has been training for years. This is because your 'training age' (the number of years you have been running) is lower and you have more room for advancement. However, there will be a point where every runner's performance will begin to decline as a consequence of

> I ran my first marathon – the London – in 1984 at the age of 23 and completed it in 4 hours 35 minutes. Twenty years later, I ran the race again, aged 43 – and finished in exactly the same time. It just goes to show that getting older doesn't necessarily mean getting slower.
>
> Cathy

ageing, regardless of when they started or how long they've run. This can be hard to accept, but setting yourself new and different goals can help you to continue enjoying running. Age group categories in races are one way of putting your performance in perspective. There are also age-adjusted tables which enable you to see what is a 'good' time for various ages (see scoremyrun.com).

When can you expect this decline to happen? In one study of more than 600,000 marathon and half-marathon runners, researchers found that biological ageing processes affected performance from the age of 54. However, the initial effects were only slight.

Running and the menopause

The menopause signals the end of reproductive potential – there is no longer enough of the hormones oestrogen and progesterone to facilitate conception. For many women, this has far greater significance than a mere biological transition. It marks the turning of the corner, the slippery slope towards old age, the passing of femininity. However you see it, you may find that running can help temper the storm.

Many female runners claim that running has been their 'lifeline' through menopause, helping to mitigate the effects, such as hormonal and mood fluctuations, weight gain and depression. In a Melpomene Institute survey more than three-quarters of the respondents said that running had a positive effect on their experience of the menopause. Meanwhile, a study of menopausal women in the *Journal of Advanced Nursing* found that a year-long exercise programme helped reduce the severity of common symptoms (e.g. hot flushes and mood swings).

Many women complain of weight gain during the menopause (research from New York found an average weight gain of 2–2.5kg over the first three years). But in a University of Pittsburgh study of 535 women who were randomly assigned to a diet-and-exercise programme or to simple weigh-ins, twice as many of those who did not exercise had gained an average of 2.35kg four and a half years later (the exercisers hadn't put on a gram). Keep on running and you may not have to battle against middle-age spread.

Safeguarding your health

Running – or aerobic exercise – is arguably even more important in protecting your health post-menopause. There are two main reasons: heart and bone health.

Under the age of 50, men are at greater risk of coronary heart disease than women but the gap closes once a woman has undergone the menopause. This is because of plummeting levels of oestrogen, which protects the heart. In post-menopausal women, the lack of oestrogen can start to affect endothelial function (the endothelium is the blood-vessel lining) as soon as three months after menopause.

Running can also help you slow the rate of bone loss post-menopause. Peak bone mass – your maximum amount of bone – happens around the age of 20 (bone growth continues a little longer for men), and from around the age of 35 bone mass declines by 0.75–1 per cent per year until menopause. In the five years following menopause, bone density can drop as much as 2–5 per cent per year, leaving bones thinner, more fragile and susceptible to osteoporosis. One study found that inactive women over 50 were 84 per cent more likely to suffer an osteoporotic fracture than those who did weight-bearing exercise at least twice a week. Exercise will also strengthen your muscles, reducing the load on joints and bones, and enhancing balance and co-ordination, helping to prevent falls in later years.

Like most women who start running in later life, I hadn't run since school. I'd represented the East Midlands in my school days, but it wasn't until my fifties, that I finally joined a running club. It was so exciting being back on the track. My 'Kelly Holmes' moment came when my club, Cambridge Harriers, won the Kent League – I won both the 100m and 200m and came first in the triple jump. At 56 it was a highlight of my athletic career. Now 63, I no longer compete, but I still love my running and all it brings to my life.

Caroline

Risk factors for osteoporosis

Osteoporosis is known as the 'silent disease' and the first symptom is often a bone fracture. If you have any reason to think you may have low bone density, it is wise to ask your doctor for a DXA bone scan prior to beginning any exercise programme. The following are all risk factors for osteoporosis:

- Early menopause or hysterectomy
- Slight build
- Family history of the disease
- Regular use of corticosteroid drugs
- Low lifelong level of weight-bearing physical activity
- Low calcium intake
- Excessive dieting or history of eating disorders
- Smoking

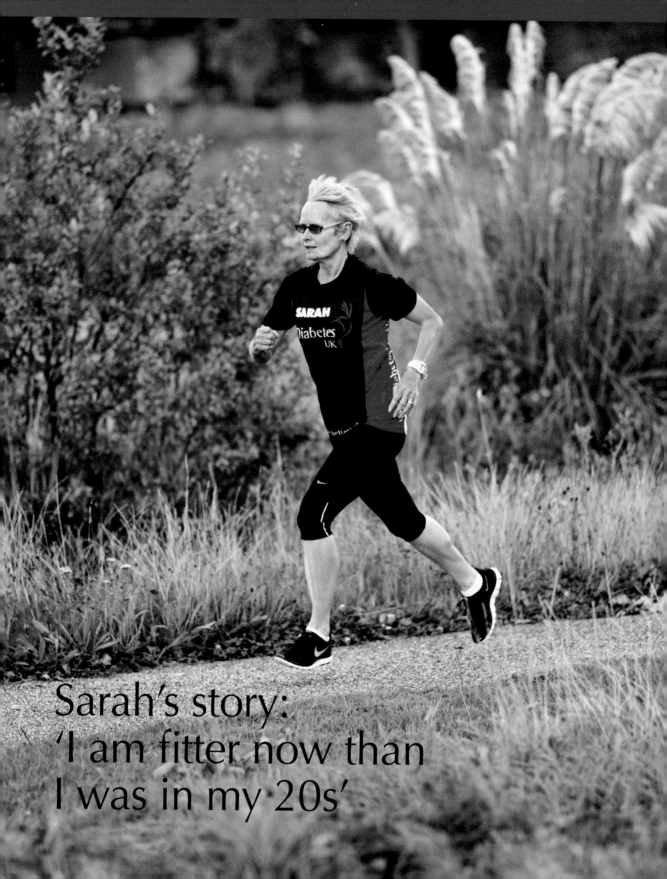

Sarah's story:
'I am fitter now than
I was in my 20s'

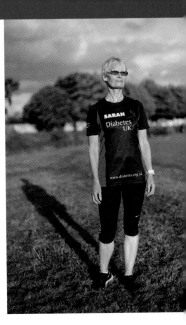

"

I was 52 when I decided to join my local running club, Hastings Runners, in order to improve my fitness and raise money for a charity challenge. I was delighted to find there were plenty of people the same age and older, enjoying running and competing in races. Although I had been moderately active before, I had not run since my school days – but the running seemed to come naturally and I found I could do quite well in my age group without really pushing myself or doing lots of training.

Running my first marathon was an incredible experience. Only months before, I would have thought it inconceivable that I could run 26.2 miles. Since then, running marathons and 'ultras' (a race that is longer than the marathon distance), especially off-road, has been one of my keenest pleasures. I've discovered that my main strength is endurance, not speed. I can keep going at a steady pace for a long time. Marathons and ultras are very different from shorter races. There is a sense of a real challenge, pushing the boundaries – and a special camaraderie among the race entrants. One of the most difficult ultras I undertook was the Lairig Ghru, a 28-mile run named after a pass in the Cairngorms in Scotland. We ran through snow and boulder fields, forests and open countryside, all surrounded by the most spectacular scenery. I felt blessed to be able to run in that landscape.

I am lucky to have joined a running club with a very strong social element – this is a fantastic bonus. There is always something to get involved with, apart from the running. When my husband died a couple of years ago, members of my running club could not have been more supportive. One couple in particular ensured that I was not moping around by inviting me to join them on their 'hash' runs (this is where a 'hare' lays a trail, including numerous false trails, for the runners to follow). We have become firm friends. Many other club members rallied round, offering me lifts to events (I do not drive), inviting me to social occasions, helping with problems in my house.

It was at this time I took on the challenge of running a marathon or ultra-marathon every month for a year, in order to raise money for Diabetes UK, as my husband had suffered from the condition. This felt like a very positive thing to do at a painful time and it helped me cope with bereavement. The challenge was dedicated to him – my thoughts were with him on every one of the challenges and, sometimes, I liked to imagine he was running beside me! I ran four marathons and 13 ultra-marathons that year - the longest being the 56-mile London to Brighton Trail Run. When it was over, my club organised a surprise party for me.

As an older woman, I find running empowering. I have been fitter during my fifties and sixties than I was in my twenties. Clearly, as time goes by, I will not be able to run as far or as fast as I have done in the past, but I hope to be able to enjoy the sociable, off-road, gentle runs for a long time to come.

"

Resources

Sam Murphy's website and blog
www.sam-murphy.co.uk

**Running technique – gait
assessment and improvement**
Natural Running
www.naturalrunning.co.uk
Get your shoes off on one of John
Woodward's educational and
inspirational Lake District-based
weekends.
Art of Running
www.theartofrunning.com
I owe a lot to Canadian running
coach Malcolm Balk for helping
me improve my running form. His
approach incorporates the Alexander
Technique and you can learn more in
his book *Master the Art of Running*.
Pose Running www.posetech.com
Learn how to rid yourself of a heel
strike with one of the pioneering
approaches to improved running
technique, Dr Nicolas Romanov's Pose
Method.
Chi Running www.chirunning.com
Chi Running marries some principles
of tai chi with a specific running
technique with a midfoot strike.
The Running School
www.runnningschool.co.uk
Have your technique assessed on a
state-of-the-art treadmill and find out
how to improve. Or send in a clip of
yourself running for online analysis.
Or come along to one of my Running
Well workshops. Find out more at
www.sam-murphy.co.uk

Physiological testing
Universities who run sport science
degree programmes frequently offer
physiological testing, such as VO_2 and
lactate threshold measurements, for
the general public. Some also offer
biomechanical assessments. Contact
your nearest university to find out.
Also try…
**The Drummond Clinic,
Maidenhead, Berkshire**
www.drummondclinic.co.uk
The Endurance Coach, Merseyside
www.theendurancecoach.com
**SportsTest, West Midlands,
South East**
www.sportstest.co.uk

Running shoes and clothing
Most UK towns now have a local
independent running shop (check the
listings in *Runner's World* magazine
or similar). Otherwise, Sweatshop has
more than 35 branches across the UK
www.sweatshop.co.uk and Up and
Running has 30 branches nationwide
www.upandrunning.co.uk
My personal favourite running store is
Run and Become in London
www.runandbecome.com for its
vast range of shoes (and kit) and
knowledgeable staff. Sports bra
specialist retailer LessBounce
www.lessbounce.com has a
comprehensive range from brands
including Sportjock, Shock Absorber,
Enell and Triumph – in sizes from AA
to J. Another great female-specific

store is SheActive www.sheactive.
co.uk, which sells all manner of
running kit, shoes and accessories
including some lesser-known brands.
Here's a rundown of some of the best
brands to check out.

Adidas www.adidas.co.uk
ASICS www.asics.co.uk
Brooks www.brooksrunning.co.uk
Gore Running Wear
www.gorerunningwear.co.uk
Helly Hansen www.hellyhansen.com
Hilly Clothing
www.hillyclothing.co.uk
Inov-8 www.inov-8.com
Mizuno www.mizunoeurope.com
New Balance
www.newbalance.co.uk
Newton www.newtonrunning.com
Nike www.nikerunning.com
Salomon www.salomon.com
Saucony www.saucony.co.uk
Skins (compression clothing)
www.skins.net
1000 mile (socks and accessories)
www.1000mile.co.uk
Vivo Barefoot
www.vivobarefoot.com

**GPS and heart rate
monitoring gadgets**
Garmin www.garmin.co.uk
Nike Plus www.nikeplus.com
Polar www.polarelectro.co.uk
Suunto www.suunto.com
Timex www.timex.co.uk

Other gadgets

Clip-on mentronome – Seiko DM-50 (widely available)

Dog leash with bungee cord – Mountain Paws Shock Absorber www.mountainpaws.co.uk

Aquajogging buoyancy belt www.aquajogger.com

Rucksacks and hydration packs

Camelbak www.camelbakuk.co.uk

Inov-8 www.inov-8.com

OMM www.theomm.com

Osprey www.ospreypacks.com

Running clubs and groups

To find a UK Athletics affiliated club, visit www.uka.org.uk

For women-only running clubs and groups try Women on the Run, which has groups across the England www.womenontherun.co.uk

To find your nearest running track, go to www.runtrackdir.com

Find a Run England group near you at www.runengland.org.uk

Find someone to run with, wherever you are, by registering with Jogging Buddy www.joggingbuddy.com

Training weekends/camps

Weekends and longer trips in the UK and abroad www.purplepatchrunning.com

Training weekends and running holidays www.runningthehighlands.com

Training camps abroad and UK weekends www.fullpotential.co.uk

Women-specific races/events

Race for Life. The UK's biggest and longest-standing female-specific running series offers beginner-friendly 5km and 10km events every summer, raising money for Cancer Research UK www.raceforlife.org

Every Woman's Series. For runners and those tempted to dip their toes in multisport adventures, a range of trail runs, aquathlons (run and swim) and duathlons (run and cycle) for women only in scenic surroundings. www.everywomansseries.co.uk

The Adidas Women's Challenge is an annual 5km in London's Hyde Park – great for your debut race. www.womenschallenge.co.uk

Pilates and yoga

Pilates UK A reference site with links to studios and classes and teacher training www.pilates.co.uk

The Pilates Foundation An acclaimed school of Pilates with accredited teachers worldwide. www.pilatesfoundation.com

Body Control Pilates A method evolved from the work of Joseph Pilates. To find accredited teachers, books and DVDs visit www.bodycontrol.co.uk

The British Wheel of Yoga is the national governing body for yoga in the UK. To find a qualified teacher or learn more about yoga visit www.bwy.org.uk

Laura Denham-Jones runs yoga and Pilates for runners workshops and classes. www.yogaforrunners.co.uk

Injury prevention and management

The Chartered Society of Physiotherapy Find a qualified physiotherapist in your area by visiting www.csp.org.uk

Sports Massage Association The UK professional body representing sports massage practitioners, with a national register of qualified therapists. www.thesma.org

The General Osteopathic Council Find a qualified osteopath at www.osteopathy.org.uk

British Chiropractic Association To find a qualified registered chiropractor in your area, visit www.chiropractic-uk.co.uk

The Society of Chiropodists and Podiatrists To find your nearest chiropodist or podiatrist, visit www.feetforlife.org

Online and written resources

Runner's World magazine www.runnersworld.co.uk

Running Fitness magazine www.runningfitnessmag.co.uk

Run247.com

Running Well by Sam Murphy and Sarah Connors (Kyle Cathie)

Marathon & Half Marathon From Start to Finish by Sam Murphy (A&C Black)

Making Sense of Barefoot Running by Lee Saxby (a free downloadable book) http://trainingclinic.vivobarefoot.com/

Master the Art of Running by Malcolm Balk (Carroll & Brown)

Index

abdominal hollowing 101
abductor stretch 96
adductor stretch 97
aerobic base 32
anaerobic/lactate threshold 17
ankle circles 43
ankle stability 100
anxiety 11, 12, 78
aqua jogging 86–7
arthritis 12
association 159
asthma 125
athletics tracks 26, 79
ATP (adenosine triphosphate) 17

babies 197
back pain 86
bags 128
barefoot running 116–17, 120
beach running 77
beetroot juice 143
blisters 121, 124
blood pressure 22
blood sugar levels 137, 139
BMI (body mass index) 22, 23, 141
    teenagers 187
BMR (basal metabolic rate) 134
body image/confidence 10–11
    teenagers 187
body scanning 55
bone density 11, 86, 142, 184
    reducing rate of bone loss 201
brain function 10, 187, 199
bras 122–3, 124, 191
breast cancer 10
breastfeeding 193, 196
breathing 51, 55, 125
    yogic 88
breathlessness 30
Bridge 101
bruised toenails 121
burnout 158

cadence 65, 77, 86
    high cadence jogging 53

measuring 50
monitoring 130
and running apps 131
caffeine 142, 178
calcium 142, 187, 200
calories
    burning 8–10, 26, 134
    cutting calorie intake 140
    daily calorie requirement 134
    and hydration 144
camps 154
canal towpaths 76
cancer 10
carbohydrates 134, 136–7, 146
    timing of eating 139-40
cardiovascular system 8, 58, 65, 78
cherry juice 143
children 184–5
chiropractors 176
cholesterol 10, 139
circadian rhythms 36
Clam 102
clothes 122–6
    `capsule' running wardrobe 124
    care of 126
    fluorescent 74, 122
    layering 122
    running after dark 172
    teenage runners 187
clubs 152, 153, 154, 155
coaches 51, 106, 154–5
coffee 142, 178
competitive running 13
compression gear 124, 126
computers 129, 130, 131
consistent training 60
contingency plans 37
conversation pace 25, 67
cooling down 26, 45
core stability 87–105, 196
    and new runners 26–30
    and posture 55
    testing 98, 100–1
    workout 101–5
costs of running 8

country parks 76
cross training 70, 84–92, 164
    aqua jogging 86–7
    elliptical trainers 85, 87
    flexibility training 93–7
    making it count 86
    and new runners 28, 29
    for performance 84, 85–6
    Pilates 29, 87, 92
    for recovery 84, 87, 175
    supportive training 84–5, 87
    yoga 29, 87, 88–91, 113
    see also cycling; swimming
Cushion squeeze 103
cycling 84, 85, 86, 87
    and new runners 26, 29

dehydration 144, 145, 199–200
depression 11, 12, 78
diaries 32, 158
diet see food and nutrition
dissociation 159
dogs 76, 156, 172
DOMS (delayed onset muscle
soreness) 178
Downward facing Dog 88

easy/recovery runs 61
eating see food and nutrition
eccentric calf raise 107
eccentric contraction 105
effort to recovery ratio 65
elasticity jumps 52
electrolyte tablets 146
elliptical trainers 85, 87
endometrial cancer 10
endorphins 12
erector spinae stretch 97
evening running 34, 36, 37
exchanges 53
excuses for not running 12–14

facilitated stretching 94
`fallback' runs 37
fartleks 63, 64, 65

fast feet 53
fat in the diet 17, 134, 138–9
    recommended intake 138
    types of fat 139
feet
    barefoot running 116–17, 120
    blisters 121
    foot care 121
    and running technique 48, 49,
        50–1
    toenails 121
    see also shoes
FIT (frequency, intensity and time)
factors 58–9, 73
fitness 12–13, 16–17
flexibility training 93–7, 111
    facilitated stretching 94
    and older runners 200
    post stretch mobility 94
    runner's stretch 95–7
    stretching properly 94
float phase 49, 50
fluorescent clothes 74, 122
food and nutrition 134–43
    daily calorie requirement 134
    disordered eating 191
    fat 134, 138–9
    protein 134, 138, 140
    race days 164
    supplements 142–3
    vitamins and minerals 141–2
    and weight loss 140–1
    see also carbohydrates
footstrike 116
frequency of running 58–9

gadgets 66, 129–31
gait 49–51
gastrocnemius stretch 96
gastrointestinal problems 178
GI (Glycaemic Index) 137
gloves 125
gluteal stretch 97
goal setting 33, 58, 59, 70
GPS watches 129, 130, 131, 161

grass, running on 26, 74, 77
gyms 34–7

haematocrit volume 17
hamstring stretch 95
hard easy rule 26, 59, 66
    and training programmes 70, 71
    and weekend running 73
hats 125
health benefits of running 8–10
    older runners 198–9
    in pregnancy 192–3
health checks 22
heart disease 10, 12, 201
heart rate 16
    and cross training 86
    monitoring 66, 67, 68–9, 77
    monitors (HRMs) 129, 131
    and warm ups 42, 43
heart rate reserve 69
heel flicks 43, 94
heel slide 102
heel strike 50–1
heel walking 43, 120
high cadence jogging 53
high intensity training 63–6
hills 26, 76, 86
    training sessions 58, 65, 66, 70
    and treadmill running 78
hip circles 43
hip flexors 95
holidays 154
HRMs (heart rate monitors) 129, 131
hydration 125, 126, 144–7
    amounts of fluid 144–5
    and hyponatraemia 147
    and race days 168
    sports drinks 145–6, 147, 178, 80
    and urinary incontinence 181
hyponatraemia 147

injuries
    ALC injuries and hormones 190–1
    common afflictions 178–81
    and cross training 64, 86–7
    dealing with 174–7
    injury prone people 176

off road running 76, 77
older runners 200
pre existing 22, 110
prevalence of 110
prevention 110–13, 184
returning to running after 161
and road running 74
and strength training 98
and treadmill running 78
intensity of running 59
interval training 59, 66, 70, 86
iron 141–2
ITP stretch 96

jackets 124, 125
joint pain 30

kinaesthetic awareness 76
knee drive 107
knee stability 100

lactate/anaerobic threshold 17
lactate threshold training 63, 64, 65
lateral stepping 104
lateral step ups 109
leg cycling drill 52
Legs Up the Wall pose 91
life expectancy 12, 199
lifestyle 8, 14, 33
Locust pose 90
long runs 61–3
lunchtime running 34, 36

mantras 159–60
marathons 137, 169, 198, 200
    training programmes 66, 72, 73
menopause 200–1
menstrual cycle 187, 190–1
MHR (maximum heart rate) 69
minimalist shoes 116–17
mitochondria 17, 198–9
mobile phones
    running data/apps 129, 131
mobility exercises 42, 43–4
morning running 34, 36
motivation 157–61
muscles

cramp 178–80
DOMS (delayed onset muscle
    soreness) 178
muscular endurance 98
muscular imbalances 87, 98
muscular pain 30
muscular strength 98
    and older runners 198–9
pelvic floor 181
and speed work 64
and warm ups 42
music 159

neuromuscular pathways 15, 85
new runners 12–13, 22–37
    attitudes to running 25, 32
    eight week programme 26–30
    first steps 25–6
    getting the habit 33–7
    health checks 22
    increasing running time 32
    measuring your progress 30–1, 67
    preparation and organisation 32,
        37
    rewards 32
    scheduling your run 34–7
    support from other people 32
    taking a break 60
    training diaries 32
    troubleshooting for 30
NSAID painkillers 177, 191
nutrition see food and nutrition

off road running 74–7, 111
older runners 14, 167, 198–203
    benefits of running for 10, 198–9
    performance 200
    post menopausal women 10, 11,
        142
omega 3 fatty acids 139, 191
1.5 mile run test 31
online running communities 152–4
osteoarthritis 14, 199
osteopaths 176, 196
osteoporosis 11, 12, 14, 141
    and menstrual disorders 191
    prevention 199

risk factors for 201
overstriding 50
overweight women 14
oxygenated blood 16–17

parkruns 167
pavements, running on 74
PBs (personal bests) 4, 33, 46, 163
pelvis
    assessing pelvic stability 100
    pelvic floor exercises 181, 196
    and running technique 48
personal trainers 106
physiotherapists 176
pick ups 53
Pigeon pose 90
Pilates 29, 87, 92
piriformis stretch 97
Plank 100, 108
plantar fascia stretch 96
PMS (premenstrual syndrome) 190
podiatrists 176
polyphenols 143
positive attitudes 32
post menopausal women 10, 11,
    142
post stretch mobility 94
posture 55
    and core stability 98
    and supportive training 87
pregnancy 86, 192–7
    benefits of running in 192–3
    body changes 193–4
    contraindications for running
        in 195
    exercise dos and don'ts for 194–5
    and foetal wellbeing 193
    running after the birth 195–7
progressive overload 58, 59
protein 134, 138, 140

Q angle 113
quadriceps stretch 95

race pace training 66, 164
races 162–9
reasons for running 4, 8–12

Reclining Big toe Hold 91
recovery 59
    and compression clothing 126
    cross training for 84, 87
    from injuries 175
    and injury prevention 11, 110
    post run snacks 139–40
    runs 61
reflective clothing 74, 122
relaxing while running 55
resistance bands 106
resisted squats 105
rest days 110–11
RHR (resting heart rate) 69
RICE protocol 174, 175
road running 74, 111
RPE (rate of perceived exertion) 67,
    68–9, 142
rucksacks 128
running apps 129, 131
running economy 16
rural areas, running in 74–7

safety 74, 76
    running alone 172–3
shoes 116–19
shorts 124
side bends 43
Side Plank 108
single leg dip 100, 108
socks 124, 125, 126
soleus stretch 96
speed/distance monitors 130
speed work 64, 66, 69, 125
    and treadmill running 78
spontaneous locomotion 12
sports bras 122–3, 124, 191
sports drinks 145–6, 147, 178, 180
sports massage 111, 113, 176
squat jumps 109
stability raises 104
stair climbers 85
stance phase 49–50, 78
static stretching 42
steady runs 61
stepover lunge 106
stitches 180

Stork 100, 103
straight leg pillar 105
strength training 84, 98–109
    core stability 98–105
    and injury prevention 111
    and muscular strength 98
    and neuromuscular pathways 105
    and new runners 26–30
    and older runners 200
    running specific workout 98,
        105–9
stress 11–12
stretching see flexibility training
strollers 197
summer clothing 126
sunglasses 126
sunscreen 126
supplements 142–3
supportive training 84–5, 87
swimming
    as a cross training activity 84, 85,
        86, 87
    health benefits compared with
running 8–10, 11
    and new runners 26, 29
    for recovery 84
swing phase 49

talk test 66
TDEE (total daily energy expenditure)
    134
technique 46–55
    ankles and feet 48, 49
    arms 48
    assessing your form 51
    awareness 55
    breathing 51, 55
    drills 52–3
    gait 49–51
    hands 48
    head 46
    heel strike 50–1
    importance of 46
    legs 48
    pelvis 48
    posture 55
    relaxing while running 55

rules for improving 52
    and running shoes 116
    shoulders 38
    torso 48
teenagers 186–9
tempo running 64, 69
threshold training
    intervals 64
    lactate 63, 64, 65
    pace 66, 67
tights 124, 126
time
    making time for running 14, 32,
        33
    time of day flow diagram 36
    and training programmes 59,
        70-3
    for new runners 26–30
    scheduling your run 34–7, 70, 73
    when to eat 138–40
toenails 121
toe walking 43, 120
tops 124, 126
trail running 74–7
training 54–81
    easy/recovery runs 61
    high intensity 63–6
    interval training 59, 66, 70, 86
    location of 74–9
    long runs 61–3
    monitoring your effort level 66–9
    new runners 32, 33–4, 37
    programmes 70–3
        5 or 10 km races 164, 165–6
        eight week programme 26–30
    race pace 66, 164
    road safety 74
    RPE levels 67, 68–9
    rules 58–60
    speed work 64, 66, 69, 125
    steady runs 61
    tailoring your training 60
    tempo running 64, 69
    and VO$_2$ max 17, 64, 66
    see also cross training; threshold
training
training partners 37

treadmill running 26, 34, 78–9
    buying a treadmill 79
    and cross training 85
    and speed/distance devices 130
    versus outdoors 78
Tree pose 89
triathlons 92
20 minute mark 32

UK Athletics' Run England 152
urinary incontinence (UI) 180–1

vests 124, 126
video feedback 55
visualisation 158, 167
vitamin D 142
vitamins and minerals 141–2
VO$_2$ max (maximal oxygen uptake)
    17, 58
    and interval training 64
    and race pace training 66

waist belts 128
walking
    as a cross training activity 86, 87
walk run strategy
    long runs 61, 63
    new runners 25–6, 32
Wall Stand 100
warm ups 42–4, 55, 111
    and flexibility training 93
    and new runners 26, 30
    and older runners 199
Warrior Lunge with a Twist 89
watches 129, 130, 131, 161
waterproof jackets 124, 125
weekend running 73
weight gain 12, 200–1
weight loss 8–10, 39, 140–1
    cutting calorie intake 140
    goal setting 33, 70
    and sports drinks 146
    teenage girls 186–7
winter clothing 125
work, running to/from 34

yoga 29, 87, 88–91, 93, 113